PUBLIC HEALTH PAPERS

No. 72

ASSESSING HEALTH WORKERS' PERFORMANCE
A Manual for Training and Supervision

ASSESSING HEALTH WORKERS' PERFORMANCE

A Manual for Training and Supervision

F. M. KATZ

Chief Scientist,
Education Evaluation,
Division of Health Manpower Development,
World Health Organization,
Geneva, Switzerland

R. SNOW

Professor of Education and Psychology,
School of Education,
Stanford University,
Stanford, CA 94305,
United States of America

WORLD HEALTH ORGANIZATION

GENEVA

1980

TYPESET IN INDIA

PRINTED IN ENGLAND

79/4622 — MACMILLAN/PITMAN—7500

CONTENTS

ACKNOWLEDGEMENTS

This publication is the product of a collaborative effort in which a number of people took part. An initial draft was prepared in the course of a consultation held in Geneva in August 1978 at which the following participants contributed to the development of the theoretical framework and procedures to be applied: Professor A. S. Elstein, USA; Dr Marion Pollock, USA; Professor T. Varagunam, Sri Lanka; Dr Janusz Wasyluk, Poland; Professor W. Wijnen, The Netherlands; Dr David Ford, WHO Regional Office for the Eastern Mediterranean; and the present authors.

Valuable criticisms of an initial draft were made by those who participated in the consultation, by Dr Karin Edström of the Division of Family Health and Dr J.-J. Guilbert of the Division of Health Manpower Development, WHO, and many others. Dr Pollock made most valuable editorial suggestions, as did Dr J. Gallagher.

The assessment instruments presented were collected in part by Professor Elstein, assisted by Dr P. Abeykoon (Sri Lanka) and Dr J. Wasyluk (Poland). We are very grateful to the authors of these instruments and to many others who provided instruments that unfortunately could not be included for lack of space.

INTRODUCTION

With training, a health worker is expected to be able to:

— immunize a child;
— diagnose and treat chickenpox;
— give nutritional advice to a pregnant woman;
— take action to control an outbreak of cholera in a community.

How can the instructor ascertain if the trainee can in fact carry out these tasks satisfactorily?

How can the instructor diagnose the trainee's difficulties so that appropriate remedial action may be taken?

Do the assessments of the trainee's performance offer sufficient guidance for future learning?

Such problems are faced by all responsible for training or supervising health workers, be they village health workers, physicians, medical assistants, nurses, or community health workers. Being responsible for helping students to acquire the necessary ability to perform specified tasks, they need to diagnose deficiencies and take appropriate action. They are required to certify various kinds of competence. Moreover, how and what they assess will determine to a large extent what is learned and how health workers function. Faced with these requirements it is essential that everyone responsible for training future health workers or supervising those in service should be able to assess performance adequately.

This is no easy task. It is essential that the assessments made are:

— valid, i.e., that they accurately assess ability to perform the tasks:
— generalizable, i.e., that, although the assessment is based only on a sample, it allows generalization to other situations;
— appropriate, i.e., that the way in which the assessment instrument is framed is suited to the function being assessed.

Unfortunately, few assessment practices to date meet these criteria. Fewer still are procedures that can provide information about a student's or practitioner's total behaviour in health care. Too often, only knowledge as to how the task should be performed is assessed. Other necessary attributes such as interpersonal skills, values, and attitudes are seldom assessed.

Similarly, most assessment practices concentrate almost entirely on measurements of ability to recall or recognize, rather than on ability to apply knowledge or to solve real-life problems. Too often, therefore, what is assessed is *not* what is really important but what is relatively easy to measure, namely, ability to memorize factual information.

Another shortcoming is that the abilities or competences assessed are often not, or only marginally, those required by the person in performing his duties as a health worker. What is assessed is not derived from a detailed analysis of job requirements. As a result, much assessment at present is irrelevant to actual health service requirements.

What, then, are the procedures that can be considered adequate for assessing the abilities of trainees and of practising health workers? The present manual sets out to assist teachers and supervisors by providing a set of guidelines on the design and use of methods for the assessment of health workers' performance. To this end the reader is invited to examine, in Chapters 1 and 2, a general approach to performance assessment. Chapter 3 offers a set of principles essential to the effective assessment of individual performance. Chapter 4 then outlines current instruments or techniques that can be applied in assessment. A sequential set of steps in preparing performance assessment is described in Chapter 5, and Chapter 6 presents examples of performance assessment procedures for specified tasks.

Part II of the manual provides the reader with some examples of instruments currently in use for the assessment of health workers' performance.

The reader not directly concerned with the design of assessment procedures may wish to concentrate on Chapters 1 and 2 and then turn directly to the examples given in Chapter 6 and in Part II of this manual.

Finally, a word of caution. This manual is intended for use by those who design, conduct, and evaluate training programmes and/or are responsible for supervising present and prospective health workers. It is not a textbook on educational measurement, a comprehensive review of assessment instruments and techniques, or an analysis of all the issues that may arise in devising, or choosing and using, appropriate assessment procedures in a particular situation. It seeks rather to provide an introduction to some alternative approaches to performance assessment and the main considerations involved in adopting any particular assessment strategy.

Part I

PRINCIPLES AND METHODS

CHAPTER 1

PERFORMANCE ASSESSMENT

What is performance assessment? Why is it so important in training health workers and in ensuring the quality of health care?

DEFINITION

Performance assessment is the measurement of an individual's ability to carry out a specified task. The use of the term "performance" is meant to focus attention on the total behaviour of a health worker, including his organization, retention, and use of specialized knowledge, as well as his attitudes and interactions with other people. It refers to the whole range of knowledge, skills, and attitudes acquired through training, as well as their organization and integration in practice.

Because of the variety of factors that go to make up human behaviour and the complex way in which they interact, it may not be useful to make arbitrary distinctions between knowledge, skills, and attitudes. Human beings anticipate. They produce mental plans to guide their functioning. They also monitor themselves to revise such plans, adapting their performance to changes in the problems they face. Performance assessments, then, must address this organizational and adaptive aspect of performance as a whole, not just the elements of performance piece by piece or step by step. This makes the task of designing performance assessments, and the task of a guide such as the present one, more complicated than they might seem at first.

The term "assessment" denotes a generalization made on the basis of an observation of events.

Since it is impossible to observe everything that is going on, assessment is always based on some kind of sampling. Hence, the aim of all assessment techniques is to systematize the way the observations are to be sampled, recorded, accumulated, and used. The goal is to increase the soundness (i.e., the accuracy and usefulness) of the generalizations derived from them.

The performance assessment of a health worker, then, may be defined as a generalization based on the observation of an individual carrying out a health care activity.

To clarify this point, it may be helpful to review some recent developments. Not long ago, most educators considered the term "evaluation" to apply mainly to the evaluation of individual students, i.e., to measures taken to judge students' academic progress and to make pass/fail or related certification decisions about them. But as "educational evaluation" grew as a field of inquiry and concerned itself more with educational programmes, institutions, and social policies, the term "assessment" began to be applied to individual students in place of "evaluation". "Assessment" had long been used in psychology to describe relatively comprehensive measurement at an individual level, as in "personality assessment". In medical education, however, such measurement remained focused on knowledge of the subject matter usually presented in university courses. More recently, terms such as "proficiencies", "competences", and "clinical skills" have come into use to refer to performance, as distinct from knowledge. To be judged competent, a health worker must be able to perform certain activities well.

Here is an example of performance assessment. One task of a health worker is to immunize a child. Performance assessment in this case requires judgement based on observation of the health worker as he carries out this task. The observation necessarily covers such points as how accurately the health worker decides on the dosage required, how he interacts with the child and parent, what follow-up activities he engages in, etc. It therefore involves assessment of a complex, interrelated set of actions in which the health worker organizes his task and adapts to the requirements of specific, often unique situations.

This example highlights the need for performance assessment techniques focusing on complex field performance. It is essential also to consider the total event rather than distinct events or elements of a sequence of behaviours. Simple distinctions between knowledge, attitudes, and skills—all elements of the performance—are therefore not useful. Nor can this total performance be assumed to equal the sum of its parts. The performance of a health worker in a complex task cannot be assessed by examining his behaviour in small segments or elements of the task.

PURPOSES

There are many reasons for performance assessment. For the student and teacher or supervisor it provides information on the quality of a given performance. In that sense, it is diagnostic, permitting the student and instructor to decide whether remedial action needs to be taken or if more remedial instruction should be given. It provides "feed-back" to both students and teacher, the latter gaining information on ways in which the programme of instruction may need revision. This *formative* process should be maintained throughout any programme of instruction or supervision. In the latter case the feedback is to the health worker and supervisor.

The purpose of *summative* assessment is to decide if an individual student should be promoted, selected, or certified (re-certified) as having the ability required to act as a health worker. At the programme level it identifies shortcomings necessitating modifications of the programme.

Thus the purposes of performance assessment fall into the four following categories:

	Formative (feedback purposes)	Summative (decision purposes)
Institutional level	Programme revision	Programme adoption
Individual level	Diagnosis of deficiencies Remedial action Self-evaluation	Selection Certification of ability Promotion

It should be apparent that formative assessment, because it provides feedback to students and health workers on their performance serves as a continuing guide to the planning of further learning opportunities.

Summative assessment provides for certification by the training institution of the ability of each student. It reaches back as an evaluation of the adequacy of aspects of the training, and forward as a means of predicting field performance.

Beyond these roles in training, performance assessment is an essential requirement for the evaluation of existing health services and thus necessary for improvements in health care. By focusing on what the health worker actually does, performance assessment provides the most direct means for measuring the quality of health care.

CHAPTER 2

A FRAMEWORK FOR PERFORMANCE ASSESSMENT

The resource to which it is usual to turn for assistance in choosing, adapting, developing, or evaluating performance assessment techniques is *educational and psychological measurement*. There are many internationally known textbooks on the subject,[1] as well as publications that define professional standards for assessment instruments, providing guidance on both the technical and the ethical issues involved in assessment.[2]

Several publications have dealt with assessment techniques applicable in the training of professional health workers. These give, however, little or no attention to performance assessment as we have defined it, concentrating instead on the methodology of examining students' knowledge in a classroom or examination centre. The methodology or instruments they describe are applicable mainly to professional students with high verbal skills and experience in traditional written examinations.

TASK ANALYSIS

In the approach to performance assessment advocated here, the first essential step is to identify the tasks of a health worker.

Health care workers face many tasks and problems in their day-to-day work and have to carry out or solve them as best they can. To assess total performance, it is helpful to break down each job into components or elements that can be more easily observed and studied. Such a breakdown helps, too, in giving better feedback to the person assessed. The feedback can focus on those job elements that the health care worker should think about, study further, or practice.

Breaking down a job into its components in this way is usually called "task analysis", a process in which different elements of a job are identified at increasing levels of specificity. This is illustrated in Fig. 1, in which an analysis of both the job and the person's behaviour in performing it is shown schematically. The total job is broken down into its several performance functions or general activities. (A, B, etc.). Each function is composed of several tasks (A1.1, A1.2, etc.), each with associated competences. This process of analysis could in theory be continued indefinitely.

An important question arises. How far should this process of differentiation be taken? For example, in the measurement of blood pressure, several performance components can be distinguished: putting the patient

---

[1] Such as: CRONBACH, L. J. *Essentials of psychological testing*, 3rd ed. New York, Harper and Row, 1970; EBEL, R. L. *Essentials of educational measurement*. Englewood Cliffs, NJ, Prentice Hall, 1972.
[2] AMERICAN PSYCHOLOGICAL ASSOCIATION. *Standards for educational and psychological tests and manuals*, Washington, DC, American Psychological Association, 1974.

at ease, placing the pressure cuff on the arm, interpreting the reading. These could be further broken down into such elements as muscular movements, special thought processes, recall of special facts, etc. The determination of the appropriate, i.e., useful, level of differentiation will vary according to the purpose of the assessment. No one level will necessarily always be the right one. In general, however, because the behaviour of human beings cannot be understood by observing separate and distinct acts, the assessment of very specific competences is often not useful. It is necessary instead to assess the complex set of interrelated actions characterizing human behaviour. Too often, a preoccupation with the detailed listing of very specific competences has resulted in meaningless data, since the essential organization and adaptive behaviour of the individual were not assessed. It is often the total sequence of actions that is important, and that is *not* simply a sum of all the separate actions involved in a task. It is for this reason that performance assessment must be concerned with more general competences.

For certain special purposes (e.g., identifying particular weaknesses of students) more detailed analysis may be necessary. However, in most cases assessment of general performance also permits the detection of critical elements at a lower level if that is needed.

Table 1 presents some major functions and constituent tasks of maternal and child health care. These are performed by several categories of community health worker—in this case, medical assistant,[1] public health midwife, trained traditional birth attendant, and community health worker.

Obviously both the functions and the job categories will differ, depending on the situation. Each task in itself contains a range of actions (components of tasks). Hence it is essential to define the total components and the competences required in order to carry out each task. This implies a detailed analysis of what the tasks will entail for each worker, and what his or her resources are for handling it. The crucial question is: "What must the worker know and be able to do to complete a given task successfully?" For instance, for the function "screening for high risk cases", three main tasks are identified. What must the worker be able to do in order to perform each of these tasks well?

The relationship between performance assessment and task analysis

A task analysis is only the first step in the development of performance assessment. It indicates what needs to be accomplished, or what the health worker needs to be able to do.

There are two main ways of obtaining the relevant information:

— Field observation of workers actually doing the task, particular

---

[1] Typically, "a health worker with eight to nine years' basic general education followed by two or three years' technical training which should enable him to recognize the most common diseases, to care for the simpler ones, to refer more complicated problems and cases to the nearest health centre or hospital, to carry out preventive measures and to promote health in his district" (*World Health*, June 1972).

FIG. 1. TASK ANALYSIS

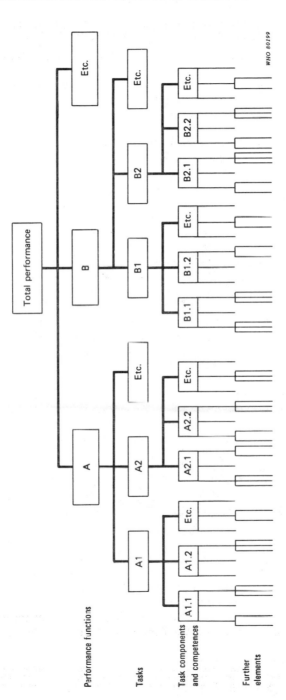

ASSESSING HEALTH WORKERS' PERFORMANCE

TABLE 1. MATERNAL AND CHILD HEALTH TASKS TO BE PERFORMED BY DIFFERENT CATEGORIES OF HEALTH PERSONNEL OUTSIDE HOSPITALS

		Category of personnel			
Function	Task	Community health worker	Trained traditional birth attendant	Medical assistant	Public health midwife
Antenatal care					
(a) Pregnancy diagnosis	__Case finding	+	+	+	+
	__Physical examination				
	__abdomen, breasts	−	+	−	+
	__gynaecological	−	−	−	+
	__Pregnancy tests	−	−	+	+
(b) Screening for, or identification of, high risk cases	__History taking	+	+	+	+
	__Physical examinations				
	__height, weight	−	+	−	+
	__abdomen	−	+	+	+
	__chest, heart	−	−	+	−
	__blood pressure	−	−	+	+
	__pelvimetry, manual	−	+	−	+
	__Laboratory testing				
	__haemoglobin	−	+	+	+
	__urinalysis	−	+	+	+
	__blood grouping	−	−	+	+
(c) Health education during pregnancy	__Child care	+	+	−	+
	__Hygiene	+	+	−	+
	__Nutrition	+	+	−	+
(d) Primary intervention during pregnancy	__Nutrition intervention (including iron supplementation)	+	+	+	+
	__Immunization (tetanus)	−	−	+	+
	__Management of cardiac failure	R	R	O	R
	__Management of moderate bleeding in early pregnancy	R	O	+	+
	__Management of incomplete abortion	R	R	R	+
	__Treatment of moderate toxaemia	−	−	−	O
	__External version of breech	−	−	−	+
	__Management of pre-eclampsia	R	R	R	O
	—Management of acute abdominal pain	R	R	O	O
	—Management of acute respiratory tract infection	O	R	+	O
	—Management of premature rupture of membranes	R	R	O	O

+ The task is normal for this category of worker.
O The worker can carry out initial observation or examinations and some treatment; referral only if necessary.
R Immediate referral to a higher level is indicated, and emergency treatment when possible.
− The task is outside the normal range of responsibilities.

attention being paid to aspects of performance that may be crucial to success or failure ("critical incidents"). Note that the organizational and attitudinal aspects of performance must be considered. In some instances the sequence of procedures or actions is important and so needs to be identified.

— Interviews with health workers, which are particularly important in order to discover the reasons for their actions.

Other procedures used are:

— work diaries
— records of actions taken and records of patients
— surveys of consumers
— patient-flow analyses
— simulations.

The information thus obtained is then used to identify the essential task components. Once these are established, it is possible to construct the necessary methodology for an assessment of performance.

Before considering this methodology, a number of principles need to be stated:

— A task analysis, no matter how comprehensive or well done, is only an abstraction of an actual job performance.
— The nature of any job will change with time and circumstances.
— Performance assessment designed to measure competence at every level of a task hierarchy is often removed from actual practice— particularly so, if the assessment is made in other than a field setting, i.e., in other than in a health service situation.
— Performance assessments made during or at the end of training are removed in time from practice. There is therefore the problem of predicting future performance in different settings.

It is important to realize that performance assessments designed to measure competence for a job or task are inescapably imperfect because of measurement errors, and because task components can never represent the total job. Many other factors such as the conditions under which the assessment is made and the personal characteristics of those being assessed (e.g., motivation and changes that are likely to occur in the job and in the person) necessarily affect the predictive capacity of any assessment.

Furthermore, measurements of performance on specific task components cannot be related closely to total performance because each of them reflects only a small portion of it. They cannot be summed up and presented as the equal of total performance because it is not simply a sum, but rather a complex of interrelated and interdependent components.

How then can any assessment be judged correct or true? How can it be validated? These are the general questions to be considered in the next chapter.

CHAPTER 3

ASSESSMENT STRATEGIES: GUIDING PRINCIPLES

The principles in the following list are intended to provide guidance on the development of assessment instruments. They can also be used by a teacher or supervisor to judge how far an instrument developed in another situation meets acceptable professional standards.

PRINCIPLE 1. RELATIVE IMPORTANCE OF ACTIVITIES

Assessment should focus upon the most critical aspects of the job as a whole. As shown earlier, a task analysis identifies an array of functions and tasks that may be assessed. Since no assessment can be truly comprehensive, the assessor must judge the relative importance of the different aspects of performance to the job as a whole. Questions to be asked include: "Is this a critical aspect of the job, i.e., is the condition for which action is needed prevalent? Would failure have a serious effect on patients, or would it seriously affect the worker's performance generally? Is it something that nearly all health care workers in a given category can be expected to have mastered? Is it a subordinate component that can be assumed to have been mastered if a superordinate component is shown to have been mastered?" From the answers to such questions, the assessor can construct a priority list. While no aspect of the job should be exempted from assessment on this basis alone, such a list gives the assessor a basis for deciding how time and effort can best be invested for the development of adequate instruments.

For example, if surveying a village for malaria prevalence is an essential function, a task of the health worker is to detect enlarged spleens by abdominal palpation. This task is a critical component of the function. The overall assessment should include a test of skill in such detection. An assessment that does not include such a test will fail to ensure that health workers can satisfactorily perform the activity of surveying a village for the prevalence of malaria.

PRINCIPLE 2. PRACTICABILITY AND COST-EFFECTIVENESS

Assessment techniques should be chosen that are practical and yield the greatest useful information for the least cost in time and money. If a performance assessment (however ideal in conception) is very costly or takes too much time, it is not appropriate and hence should not be used. An assessment must be practicable in a particular situation. Hence the assessor may have to discard a first-rate plan that is too costly, or for which the technology is lacking, and use a less than perfect plan that can be implemented.

Cost must always be considered. The assessor should concentrate on the most important aspects of performance and seek to develop cheap and convenient methods. If this is kept in mind, the limited resources for performance assessment can be spread, thereby increasing the representativeness of the assessment.

An example is provided by some medical schools in developing countries, which use electronic simulators that reproduce with high fidelity the sounds heard in diseased hearts. These elegant instruments can assess the auscultatory skills of students, but are very expensive. The money spent on such gadgets could very well be used to develop ways of measuring other important functions, and the ability to detect deviations of heart sounds could be tested more cheaply with simple audiotapes, phonograph records, or actual patients.

PRINCIPLE 3. REPRESENTATIVENESS AND CONTENT VALIDITY

The performances assessed should represent the full range of competences for the functions and tasks demanded by the job. Most functions and tasks require particular knowledge, certain skills (including interpersonal skills), practical decision-making, and positive attitudes. All of these should be assessed. The assessor should guard against the temptation to measure what is relatively easy to measure, and at all times be concerned with the totality of behaviours and skills required to perform a task well.

As far as possible the setting in which assessment is made should resemble the real work situation. In practice, however, all assessments will include some artificial elements. This is often necessary and sometimes even desirable, since in a simulated situation conditions can be controlled and feedback given.

Assuming that a task analysis has provided a definition of the content of the job, it is essential for the assessment techniques used to obtain samples that are representative of every aspect of this content (N.B., it is always necessary to sample). If the assessment is designed to yield such representative samples it has "content validity", no important function or task will be omitted, and none will be given weight out of proportion to the job.

An adequate assessment plan is often a compromise between the three principles just reviewed.

PRINCIPLE 4. MULTIPLE MEASUREMENT

The most important and critical aspects of performance should be assessed by more than one method or approach. Because the functions of health workers are so varied and complex, no single formula or strategy for performance assessment can adequately assess all of them. Different combinations of knowledge, technical skills, decision-making and problem-solving capabilities, and attitudes will be required, depending on the future functions and tasks of the worker concerned. A variety of instruments must therefore be used and the best combination will depend on the functions to be assessed and the resources of the evaluator.

Even though one way to ensure accurate measurement is to use more than one method, *every* method has some shortcomings. If two methods are used to measure one performance function, such weaknesses may cancel one another out. When different means of measurement agree despite different weaknesses, confidence in the assessment is increased.

A good example of this principle is provided by the assessment of a health worker's ability to communicate with patients. This can be assessed, using a suitable checklist as a guide, by observing him as he talks with a patient. It can also be checked with the patient after the health worker has talked with him. When the conclusions agree, one can be reasonably confident of their validity. In order to ascertain whether successful communication between health worker and patient had taken place, the patient's subsequent behaviour might also be observed to see whether his talk with the health worker had produced the desired effect.

PRINCIPLE 5.   PREDICTIVE VALIDITY

Performance assessment should be predictive of future performances of the same task or function. As noted above, representativeness of sampling ensures the *content validity* of the assessment, and multiple measurement of important functions heightens the validity of the means employed. But validity is not a "property" that an assessment instrument "possesses" in itself. About any form of measurement, one question must always be asked: "Valid for what purpose?" Predictive validity is a third aspect of correctness in measurement.

When the performance of students or health workers is assessed, the teacher or supervisor is concerned ultimately with how they will perform in similar situations later on. As far as possible, assessment should predict future performance.

It is realized, as has already been pointed out, that assessments made during or at the end of training may not correlate well with later performance. Conditions change and so do people, and the limitations of assessment as regards prediction of future behaviour must be recognized.

Moreover, an assessment can only measure whether a health worker *can* do something. It cannot tell us that he *will* do it, or will perform in the same manner subsequently. For example, if a student or health worker knows he is being assessed in his work by his supervisor, he will naturally want to perform at his best. Also, students are often assessed on only one problem or case at a time and can give it their undivided attention. In practice, however, a health worker usually has to deal with several problems simultaneously. The mental effort of managing several patients in quick succession is likely to lead to occasional slips and errors that might not occur with only one patient and plenty of time. In this respect, therefore, assessment situations are often "artificial".

Generally an accurate assessment of a student reflects the potential upper limits of his future performance of a similar task.

PRINCIPLE 6. RELIABILITY

A performance assessment should have stability and internal consistency. In addition to validity, correct assessment requires precision in measurement. This aspect is usually referred to as "reliability". One indication of reliability is internal consistency, i.e., how well subscores on similar items within, for example, a test or rating scale agree with one another. Stability, the second requisite for reliability, is demonstrated when assessments of the same students for the same task at two different times agree with one another.

When observations are used in assessments of this sort, reliability is established on the basis of agreement between the findings of the observers or judges concerned. A related concept is "objectivity", that is, that the assessment should not be unduly influenced by the personal biases of the observer or judge.

In recent years, the quest for objectivity, and hence for greater reliability, in medical education has led to the increased use of multiple-choice examinations in which the correct answer or combination of answers is determined by a panel of experts before the test is administered.

But there are important aspects of a health worker's performance that cannot and should not be assessed with such tests. In fact, they have a very limited use in performance assessment. Generally, performance is better assessed by so-called subjective measurements. For example, ratings of a worker's effectiveness in relating to patients can be easily and conveniently obtained from the patients themselves. A series of patients may be asked questions such as "Did you understand the directions the doctor gave you?" or "Did you feel comfortable talking with that nurse?" Their replies will unquestionably be subjective for they depend upon perceptions and personal feelings. Yet to obtain a convenient, inexpensive, and feasible assessment of a worker's interpersonal skills, this may be a satisfactory technique. If the statements of a patient agree in general with those of the other patients questioned, this suggests that the assessment is reliable.

Here a word of caution is needed about the distinction frequently made between "subjective" and "objective". Objectivity is simply a matter of reliability, which in turn can only be understood in terms of generalizability. Assessments are always subjective in that they involve judgement. Objectivity is established when, for the same performance, similar results are obtained with different observers, or different items, or scales or measures, and it is thus possible to generalize from one observation or measurement to another.

Although reliability is desirable, it should not be such an overriding principle of assessment as to blind one to the need to assess other aspects of performance that, by their very nature, call for more personal, subjective means of measurement. And, while agreement between raters is important, variation among them, whether they are teachers or patients, may tell us something about the natural variability of a student's performance rather than reflect "subjectivity" or "error" in measurement. If an assessment of a student's performance varies with time, we also need to know how much of the variation is actually due to changes in competence and how much to other, undetermined factors in the measurement. The "trade-off" between more objective and more subjective measurement should be considered each time in the light of the aspect of performance to be assessed.

PRINCIPLE 7. INEVITABLE COMPROMISES

The purpose of assessment should be considered when choosing among assessment techniques. A compromise between relative importance, cost-effectiveness, and content validity has already been noted in connexion with Principles 1, 2, and 3. The compromise, or "trade-off", between more objective and more subjective approaches to measurement has also been noted. Many such compromises are inevitable in any assessment plan. There is a particular need to compromise between reliability and validity— this is often called the "band-width fidelity" dilemma. To increase the reliability, i.e., the fidelity or accuracy, with which any function or competence is measured, the length of the assessment instrument is increased, thus permitting additional observations. However, this entails a reduction in the number of observations of other critical functions or competences. The band-width fidelity of the instrument has been reduced and thus the content validity and possibly also the predictive validity of the assessment.

Broad band-width is needed in assessments of health care functions because of the wide spectrum of responsibilities and activities that is usually involved. Consequently, it is necessary to compromise to some extent on the fidelity with which any one function is assessed, otherwise the length of the instrument becomes a problem. Of course, different purposes of assessment will demand different kinds of band-width compromise.

PRINCIPLE 8. ASSESSMENT AS A GUIDE TO LEARNING

Performance assessment procedures should provide a guide to student learning. Since what and how a student learns will be markedly influenced by how he is assessed, it is essential that the form or procedures used are clearly related to learning requirements. In terms of content, this means that if the assessment concentrates on health care competences, students are more likely to become concerned with health care practices. If the assessment focuses on recall of factual information, the student is likely to concentrate on learning facts or storing information.

But it is not only the content but also the process used that is important. For instance, the exclusive and constant use of multiple-choice tests, or of essays, or of short-answer tests can influence students to learn selectively only what is assessable by a particular form of examination.

———————

CHAPTER 4

ASSESSMENT TECHNIQUES

TECHNIQUES USED IN CONVENTIONAL EXAMINATIONS

The traditional ways of assessing student knowledge in most educational programmes for health personnel commonly include the following types of test:

— essays
— short-answer (completion) tests
— oral tests
— multiple-choice tests.

There are many publications that review the different techniques employed, the construction of the tests, and the interpretation of the results.[1] Such tests can play an important role in performance assessment if properly used as part of a more general assessment.

Each has some strengths and weaknesses. For instance, the essay can be used to measure the student's ability to organize, integrate, or synthesize information. It can also be used more effectively than short-answer or multiple-choice tests to measure originality or innovative approaches to problems. The multiple-choice test is more likely than the essay to lead to adequate sampling of factual information and to inter-examiner consistency in analysis or scoring.

All these approaches concentrate mainly on assessment of knowledge and often on memory (recall and recognition) of information. Apart from the oral examination, they obviously are suitable only for trainees with a high level of literacy.

Because multiple-choice tests have recently gained in popularity and are increasingly used in the assessment of students in the health professions in many parts of the world, an additional comment seems appropriate.

The multiple-choice form of assessment is attractive in that it has the advantage of objectivity in marking. The tests are relatively easy to score and lend themselves to mechanical scoring and analysis, thus apparently saving valuable time for teachers and supervisors. However, the papers take more time to set than do those for essays, short-answer tests, or oral tests. The time is thus merely shifted from test-scoring to test-setting, at least if the setting is done properly (and a badly designed test has no merit at all). Caution is therefore indicated in the use of this technique. As with all assessment, the assessor must be clear as to *why* he wants to assess, *what* he wants to measure, and *who* the candidates are.

---

[1] See, for example: CHARVAT, J. ET AL. *A review of the nature and uses of examinations in medical education.* Geneva, World Health Organisation, 1968 (Public Health Papers, No. 36); GUILBERT, J. J. *Educational handbook for health personnel.* Geneva, World Health Organization, 1968 (WHO Offset Publication No. 35).

In general, none of these techniques yields valid assessments of field performance. Although a certain minimum of reliability is required of any means of assessment, the crucial requirement is *validity*. This is emphasized here because too often in recent times the emphasis has been on obtaining greater reliability and objectivity, often to the detriment of validity. As a general rule, a test is worthless, however great its reliability, however "objective" it appears to be, if it does not measure abilities important in enabling the health worker to carry out the health care functions for which he is responsible.

It is therefore essential to use or develop other approaches that offer advantages in validity without significant losses in reliability. For example, the best way of finding out whether a health worker can take the history of a woman in the second trimester of pregnancy is *not* to set a series of multiple-choice questions asking, in effect, what are the major points to be covered in such a history. Instead, the teacher or supervisor should develop a check-list of these points and use it while directly observing a series of student-patient encounters. In this case it is the student's actual performance with patients that is assessed, not just what the student recognizes as correct among a set of alternative actions laid before him. Direct observation like this is often a valid means of measuring the student's competence in taking the history, and the use of a check-list increases reliability in that it structures the observer's ratings (thus increasing the potential for inter-observer agreement).

A case can also be made for oral examinations in the field. During or immediately following an actual performance, an observer can ask questions (e.g., "Why did you do . . .?" "What would you have done if . . .?" etc.) to assess dynamic organization and use of knowledge in real problem-solving situations. Such assessments may lack reliability for some purposes, but they can provide a rich and representative description of knowledge being applied. Oral questions that require only reproduction by rote of memorized knowledge have no place in field assessment. They should be used only in training, if at all.

FIELD OBSERVATION: CHECK-LISTS AND RATING SCALES

The most obvious and essential procedure in performance assessment is careful observation of a health worker in an actual service or field setting. There can be no substitute for such observation in actual practice. It is the most direct, timely, and inexpensive means of performance assessment.

The observations have to be sound and accurate, which is to say that they must have validity and reliability. It is the task of the assessor to organize observations so that data will be collected systematically and will be comparable among different observers. For this, the observers will need guidance in the form of check-lists and rating scales, which they must be trained to use.

Check-lists require the observer to judge whether certain behaviour has taken place (for examples, see Part II of this manual). They can be used most effectively when components of performance can be specified in detail. It is then possible for the observer simply to note whether the prescribed behaviour has taken place or not. For example, a check-list could be used in observing the activities of a health worker taking blood pressure or giving an injection. The actual physical or psychomotor skills involved can be fairly precisely stated.

Carefully prepared check-lists can be used, however, for more complex kinds of performance (see Part II).

In many cases, the observations must cover factors other than whether something was done or not. One such factor is sequence. Some actions must be performed in a certain sequence if a given task is to be done competently. Most laboratory procedures, and some physical examinations, fall into this category. Often, however, the fixed sequence prescribed by some instructors is not only unnecessary but positively harmful. For instance, in medical history-taking, strict adherence to a routine would be ineffective and inefficient. Hence a fixed sequence of actions should not be required or figure in assessment, unless it is essential to the task.

There are other aspects of performance that do not lend themselves to assessment by check-list. For example, the important aspect known as "attitude" or "style" is part of all interactions between health workers and others—patients, village elders, fellow members of the health team, etc.— and thus needs to be included in performance assessment for many functions. Interaction with others, or personal style, can be observed and assessed by means of a check-list, but not easily. A "correct" list of acts or components of behaviour can rarely be prescribed in this connexion. Rather, the assessor-observer recognizes that, while a certain sequence of behaviour may seem to fit the situation well and leads to the desired outcome, another health worker might have used an entirely different sequence and arrived at the same effect. Rating scales are more likely to provide a better record of such aspects of performance than check-lists. The observer can take informal notes as he observes the health worker in the interpersonal transactions of the task. He will especially note critical exchanges that reflect different personal styles or attitudes. Later, the observer will sum up his impressions in ratings on one or more scales. His notes ought to provide a justification for the rating as well as a basis for more detailed feedback to the worker or trainee.

A rating scale requires judgements by the observer on how well the performance meets specified criteria. This is particularly useful when there is no set routine, but a number of alternatives, or when the health worker is required to adapt to local characteristics and variations.

In the case of workers taking blood pressures, for example, a rating scale could be used to assess how they interact with patients and whether they succeed in putting them at their ease. Another case in which a rating scale would be more appropriate than a check-list is the assessment of a health worker's performance in persuading village elders to change a sanitation practice.

Whether to use a check-list or a rating scale is often a matter of personal choice, and no strict guideline in the matter can be laid down. For many aspects of performance either would serve. In general, however, check-lists serve assessment especially well when the components of performance can be specified in detail and follow a routine. Performances for which there is no single routine, but a number of alternatives, or which require the health worker to adapt to local characteristics and variations, are probably better served by rating scales.

Finally, although it has been stated that observation in actual field conditions is undoubtedly the preferable approach in performance assessment, the means described above—check-lists and rating scales—are also applicable to assessments in other settings, e.g., in classrooms, examination centres, etc. In certain cases, the simulation of conditions encountered in practice may have some advantages.

SIMULATION

Many aspects of health care may be simulated for assessment purposes. Simulation has the advantage of approximating reality while retaining the standardized character of the traditional examination, and it avoids some of the disadvantages of working with patients.

For example, to assess ability in diagnostic problem-solving and decision-making, the thought processes and intermediate judgements of the trainee should be investigated. The assessment should concern itself with ability to obtain information from patients, problem formulation and hypothesis generation, data interpretation, integrative diagnostic judgement, and choosing between alternative courses of action. The observation of encounters with patients has immediate appeal and high content validity, but using patients may be less desirable than using specially designed simulations. These can include written case-histories and "paper-and-pencil" patient management problems, patient simulation, and oral examinations in which an assessor or instructor plays the part of the patient and evaluates the student's performance at the same time. In such encounters, planning and reasoning can be displayed more clearly and openly than is usually possible with real patients. The student can be asked to explain the reasons for a particular action, either orally or in writing, and can discuss strategic alternatives and doubts, indicate points of uncertainty or confusion, and state why a particular decision was taken. By contrast, in typical interactions with patients, the thought processes underlying clinical decisions are not displayed and the student or health care worker is understandably reluctant to show doubt or uncertainty. For performance assessments, therefore, some simulations are of greater content validity than clinical encounters.

There is another argument for simulation. Assessment validity will generally be increased by more extensive sampling of relevant events. But the time available for assessment is limited. With paper simulation less time is usually spent per case than with actual patients, and a wider sampling of different kinds of cases is possible. For this reason also, the use of simulations may have greater content validity than the use of a series of unselected patients, although the latter would appear at first sight to be more valid.

INTERVIEWS

Often the assessment of performance requires not only systematic observation of the health worker in a field situation or simulated practice setting, but much useful information can also be gained from interviews with persons with whom the worker has been in contact in the course of his work, e.g., patients, team-members, etc.

Here again it is important to be systematic. Guides on interviewing should be prepared, and those conducting interviews should be trained. It is only in this way that some degree of consistency can be attained.

A special form of interview is the oral examination cited earlier as one of the conventional techniques of assessment. The use of oral examinations has become less popular as evidence has accumulated of their low reliability and doubtful content validity. In addition, they are time-consuming. However, an oral test—i.e., a careful interview—can often make an important contribution to performance assessment. It may often be easier to ask the trainee or health worker for an explanation, or comments on alternative actions, than to use techniques such as short answer or multiple-choice examinations.

PERFORMANCE PROFILES

Once information has been collected by means of observations in the field or a simulated practice setting, using check-lists, rating scales, observation schedules, and conventional examination techniques where appropriate, it is necessary to summarize the findings and pronounce on the performance.

Data obtained from several assessments are not easy to combine. The widespread practice of adding together scores for different performances to arrive at a single general judgement cannot be recommended. The competent health worker would not add together a patient's temperature and blood pressure readings to constitute a general health index. The competent assessor avoids the analogous practice of averaging performance data.

Different assessment purposes call for different treatments of the data. A generally useful practice is to construct a performance profile, which shows a *pattern* of performance across different aspects of the job, and for different workers, without recourse to total scores.

This profile is based on a rating scale. In the following example, a five-point scale is used with "unacceptable" and "acceptable" as the extremes. In addition, another point is prescribed as the "minimum acceptable performance standard", usually on the basis of an arbitrary decision that should be taken before the profile is used. It can be determined by identifying essential tasks or task components that must be satisfactorily accomplished, or by the reverse process, i.e., by identifying behaviour incompatible with an acceptable performance. In either case, a rating less than that specified is unacceptable.

Hypothetical profiles for two health workers, constructed at the level of function, are shown below (Fig. 2). The profiles represent the antenatal care functions in the maternal and child health matrix. For each function the scores of two independent observers are shown. Each observer has used a check-list to assess performance on each of the tasks and task components and then recorded a rating on a continuous scale for each function. The two observers' ratings agree for the most part, but diverge occasionally, particularly for health worker 2. Note that a minimum performance standard has been stipulated.

FIG. 2. PERFORMANCE PROFILES

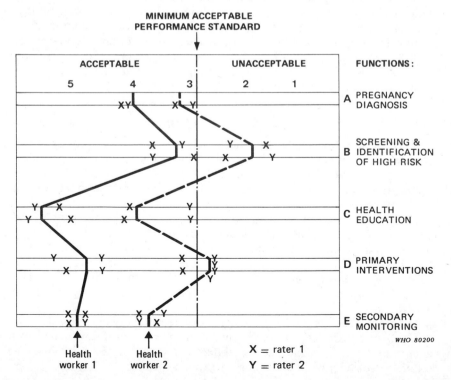

The performance of health worker 1 in all functions is judged acceptable by both observers, but some weakness is noted in "Screening and identification of high risk". On noting this, a teacher, student, supervisor, or worker could consult the check-list for this function to find out which performance components needed to be strengthened. Health worker 2 shows inadequate performance on two functions, but the judges disagree somewhat. Again, the check-lists for these functions can be consulted to decide what the worker must do to improve his performance.

Profile patterns may also have implications for the training programme. Suppose that a number of workers in one place showed profiles similar to those of workers 1 and 2. A teacher or supervisor might then conclude that training for function B—"Screening and identification of high risk"— should be revised.

CHAPTER 5

PLANNING ASSESSMENT STRATEGIES AND PROCEDURES

The material in the previous chapter can be restated as a series of steps for planning a performance assessment strategy and procedure. All the steps are necessary, but how they are carried out and the order in which they are taken will vary.

Sometimes the assessor finds that steps 1–4 have already been taken; they are prerequisites to assessment, and to some extent require different skills and knowledge than do the later steps. When they have not been taken and the necessary expertise is not available, the assessor must carry them out.

Steps 5–13 are the principal responsibility of the assessor, i.e., the person primarily concerned with the design and use of performance assessment. In addition, he has to ensure that steps 14–15 are planned and responsibilities for them assigned. Steps 14–15 are the most important follow-up steps since they involve specialized expertise. Considerable expenditure of effort and additional manpower resources (consultants) may be required.

PREREQUISITES

Steps 1–4

The purpose of these procedures is to ensure that job functions and tasks are identified. These are sometimes already identified and available from the Ministry of Health or can be inferred from the institutional objectives of the training programme. Where they are not available, the task of identifying them falls to those responsible for designing performance evaluation.

1. Identify job(s) for which performance assessment is needed and which meet priority health needs.

2. Conduct a job analysis to identify general activities or functions; divide these further into tasks and task components, using some combination of expert judgement, observation of job performance, interviews with workers known to be effective on the job, and other procedures that permit identification of job elements.

3. Identify the job functions and tasks that are most critical for health care, and thus for job success, and that are feasible.

4. Identify all other job functions and tasks that will be assessed.

PLANNING THE ASSESSMENT PROCEDURES

Steps 5—13

The purpose is to provide those responsible for training or supervision with valid and reliable techniques for performance assessment. The techniques will give appropriate guidance to students or health workers on what is expected of them.

5. Decide the levels at which assessment will be made—functions, tasks, and/or task components—taking into account the relative importance of the tasks and the cost of assessment.

6. Choose the approaches and techniques that will be used to measure performance in each function and task. Decide which performances, if any, need multiple measurement.

7. Select all required instruments (procedures) or, where necessary, design them.

8. Arrange for a review of these instruments by other experts who know the jobs to be assessed, as well as the conditions in which the instruments are to be used, and have some knowledge of performance assessment. This review should check the representativeness (content validity) of the set of instruments and whether the measurements chosen are suitable. Revise or adjust as necessary.

9. Conduct a pilot study of the instruments. This should include an estimation of reliability, and checks on whether the set of instruments is practicable and feasible, whether the instructions are adequate for the health care workers being assessed, whether those who will use them are adequately trained and instructed, and whether there are other factors that could affect the assessment strategy. If possible, check also how far multiple measures of a function or task agree with each other.

10. Revise the provisional assessment instruments as needed, on the basis of the results of the pilot study and any other reviews. Adopt the final assessment plan.

11. Plan the data-recording procedures. Design the standard performance profile record that will be used to summarize results for each health care worker.

12. If indicated, establish minimum acceptable performance standards for each function or task to be assessed. This calls for the judgement of experts such as those referred to in step 8. The standards might in fact be established as part of step 8. How step 12 is carried out will depend on local conditions and the specific purposes of the performance assessment.

13. When indicated and possible, arrange for a study of the predictive validity of the assessment instrument. Sometimes this step can be included in the pilot study carried out as part of step 9, or a separate pilot study may be required. Occasionally, a predictive validity study can be made in the course of the assessment itself.

FOLLOW-UP

Steps 14–15

Follow-up activities are often neglected, but they are an important part of planning and adopting an assessment process. It is only through such activities that an assessor can satisfy himself and others that the process is adequate and is achieving the desired results. They constitute an evaluation of the assessment procedure itself.

14. Design a procedure to monitor the adequacy—including the acceptability—of the assessment procedures. Useful sources of information are other teachers, supervisors, other assessment experts, observers, and health workers.

15. As assessment data accumulate, examine performance profiles for each job, function, or task. From these, a distribution of profiles can be made that allows a revision of the minimum standards established in step 12, if this is necessary.

SELECTION OF ASSESSMENT PROCEDURES BY USERS

The development of a methodology for performance assessment is obviously the task of specialists who have had some special training in educational measurement. However, every teacher or supervisor of health personnel will need to engage in performance assessment as an essential part of his or her duties. The following steps are recommended for the non-specialist concerned with application, i.e., the use of assessment procedures already developed.

Prerequisite steps

These are the same as those suggested for planning assessment procedures. Any user of performance assessment will need to have identified the functions and tasks for which his students are being trained or that the health worker who is being supervised must carry out. Hence the user must first proceed in accordance with steps 1–4 outlined above.

Process of selection

The selection of appropriate procedures will involve:

1. Identification and listing of all functions, tasks, and task components to be assessed by the procedures.

2. A review of techniques and instruments already being used, whether locally or in other settings (examples, which will be updated from time to time, will be found in Part II of this manual).

3. Selection of the most appropriate techniques on the basis of the pilot study. Examination of any data available for predictive validity and reliability.

4. A review of the selected procedures by colleagues familiar with the jobs to be assessed and by students and health workers who are to be assessed.

5. Organization of a pilot study (see step 9 above).

6. Revision of the tentative procedures on the basis of the results of the pilot study.

Interpretation

The user of any assessment procedure ultimately has to answer two questions:

1. Can the health worker perform the specific function?
2. Can the health worker be certified as competent?

If the assessment uses the approach suggested here, i.e., breaking down the total job into functions and their component tasks, both questions are in principle the same. In each case total competence is judged on the basis of information about the component parts of a function. *The ultimate judgement remains subjective and should be made by experienced practitioners.* The validity of the judgement will be enhanced if the following principles are borne in mind:

1. The judgement depends on the purpose of the assessment. If the purpose is to diagnose the student's strengths and weaknesses in order to help him in his learning, it is best to draw up a profile of his performance, so that he can see where he needs to improve.

2. Total performance cannot be judged simply by adding up the scores recorded in tests of its component parts. The total performance has to be observed by the assessor and when he decides intuitively that it is "not up to the mark" he should identify the shortcomings in order to give useful feedback to the student.

3. When assessing the performance as a whole, adequate weight should be given to the more important components. For example, if a student does not prescribe morphine for acute left heart failure, he cannot be certified as competent to manage cardiac emergencies, however well he scores in the other aspects of management of cardiac emergencies.

4. When information on the predictive validity of the instruments of assessment is available, it should be taken into consideration. Particular reliance should be placed on data obtained through instruments known to be of high predictive validity.

CHAPTER 6

TWO EXAMPLES OF PERFORMANCE ASSESSMENT PROCEDURES

The two following examples are given to illustrate the procedures outlined in the previous chapter.[1]

The function or general activity to be assessed is part of antenatal care, more specifically "screening for or identifying high-risk cases". The tasks are "history-taking" and "measuring blood pressure". Hence, the purpose of the assessment is to determine the competence of students or health workers to collect valid and reliable data from a pregnant woman as a prerequisite for deciding on appropriate care or management.

The decisions to be taken will necessarily vary in different situations depending on the organization of the health care system and the availability of personnel and facilities. Similarly the data collection involved will depend on the circumstances prevailing in the health care system, notably the time and facilities available to the health worker. For example, in some settings a worker may be expected to identify abnormal or potentially problematic findings and to refer them to other categories of health worker. In other settings, the collection of data is part of a set of responsibilities that include interpretation of the data, problem formulation, and deciding on management.

The specific tasks "history-taking" and "measuring blood pressure" have the following components.

1. History-taking

— obtaining sufficient data relevant to the decision to be made
— establishing communication with the patient that will be supportive to her and facilitate her responsiveness to the health worker
The abilities required thus include:
— ability to obtain essential medical-social history
— ability to record pertinent information
— ability to establish and maintain effective interaction with a patient
— ability to organize information obtained as a basis for subsequent decision-making.

2. Measuring blood pressure

This widely used procedure in epidemiology, preventive and curative medical care, and rehabilitation involves:

[1] They have been developed for this purpose by Professor A. S. Elstein, Office of Medical Education Research and Development, Michigan State University, East Lansing, MI, USA, and Dr Lauren M. Eyres, Office of Educational Research, College of Human Medicine, Michigan State University, East Lansing, MI, USA.

— obtaining the cooperation of a patient
— making an accurate reading
— assessing the reliability of the reading made
— making an initial interpretation of the results obtained.
  The abilities required thus include:
— ability to enlist the collaboration of a patient, to make her feel sufficiently relaxed and confident
— skill in carrying out the set of actions involved in the application of the cuff and the placement of the stethoscope
— ability to read pressure accurately
— ability to interpret and record the reading and judge its accuracy (reliability)
— ability to interpret the results using the standard values provided.

THE PROCEDURES

History-taking

The example given here takes the form of a rating scale to be used by trained observers. A version of this scale has been used satisfactorily in several health care settings. It was adapted by Professor A. S. Elstein and Dr L. M. Eyres from several earlier forms used mainly with nurses in prenatal clinics in the Lansing, MI, area of the USA. The forms were originally designed for evaluating a pregnant woman's health status and not for assessing a health worker's performance in taking a history. The authors added several sections to make the form more appropriate, and the section on history of previous pregnancies was substantially expanded.

The scale is thus an adaptation of several others used in different contexts. Results of studies on its validity and reliability are not yet available. It must be stressed that the scale cannot and should not be used in other settings without adaptation. Other procedures that might be used in addition to the rating scale, but are not presented here, are:
— interview of patient
— the use of patient management problems.

Measuring blood pressure

The procedures are:
— a rating scale
— check by observers of readings made.

Other possible procedures not illustrated are:
— questioning of patient
— oral assessment of description of procedure.

The rating scale is substantially revised and expanded from an examination feedback form initially developed by Dr L. M. Eyres and Dr E. Grandblatt for use in a second-year physical diagnosis course at the College of Human Medicine, Michigan State University. The trainees in this case are medical students learning physical examination skills; their assessors are physicians.

THE RATING FORMS

History-taking

This rating form provides for the assessment of three aspects of performance.

1. Was each question on the history form asked? A score of zero (0) means a question was omitted.

2. Was the question asked in such a way that the patient could easily understand it? To assess this, the assessor could exercise his or her clinical judgement or, following the examination, the patient could be asked whether certain terms or sentences used by the student examiner were understood by her, or how she understood what was being said to her. A score of one (1) should be given to questions that are poorly phrased.

3. If a positive response to a question was obtained, were appropriate additional questions asked to gather pertinent details of the situation? Did the student expand on the subject appropriately when a positive response was obtained? Depending on the quality of this response, a score of 2, 3, or 4 is to be assigned.

EVALUATION OF HISTORY-TAKING FOR PRENATAL HEALTH CARE BY MATERNAL AND CHILD HEALTH TRAINEE

Name of patient _____

Name of trainee _____

Name of evaluator _____

Program _____

Site _____

Date _____

Rating scale

0 = Omitted or forgot to expand on question

1 = Basic technique needs review; question poorly phrased

2 = Understands basic technique, but needs more practice

3 = Speed, style, and manner good

4 = Speed, style, and manner excellent

	Rating				
A. Past obstetrical history					
1. Menarche	0	1	2	3	4
2. Menstrual cycle,_____ days					
Varies,_____to_____days	0	1	2	3	4
3. Gravida_____	0	1	2	3	4
4. Abortion/miscarriage	0	1	2	3	4
5. Live children, number_____	0	1	2	3	4
6. Stillbirths, number_____	0	1	2	3	4
7. Previous pregnancies,	0	1	2	3	4
Fill out separate form for each					
B. Current pregnancy					
1. Contraception	0	1	2	3	4
Type _____					
Date discontinued _____					
2. Last menstrual period (LMP)	0	1	2	3	4
3. Previous menstrual period (PMP)	0	1	2	3	4
4. Quickening	0	1	2	3	4
5. Symptoms since LMP					
(a) Nausea and vomiting, indigestion	0	1	2	3	4
(b) Constipation	0	1	2	3	4
(c) Vaginal bleeding or discharge	0	1	2	3	4
(d) Abdominal pain	0	1	2	3	4
(e) Infection	0	1	2	3	4
(f) Radiological examination	0	1	2	3	4
(g) Medications, current and since LMP	0	1	2	3	4
(h) Other[1]	0	1	2	3	4
C. Past medical history					
Vascular	0	1	2	3	4
Viral infections	0	1	2	3	4
Heart, rheumatic fever	0	1	2	3	4
Hypertension	0	1	2	3	4
Diabetes	0	1	2	3	4
Kidney, bladder	0	1	2	3	4
Jaundice, transfusion	0	1	2	3	4
Thyroid disease	0	1	2	3	4
Venereal infection	0	1	2	3	4
Accidents, surgery	0	1	2	3	4
Other[1]	0	1	2	3	4
D. Family history					
Diabetes	0	1	2	3	4
Hypertension	0	1	2	3	4
Cancer	0	1	2	3	4
Health of infant's father	0	1	2	3	4
Inherited illness	0	1	2	3	4
Anomalies, twins	0	1	2	3	4
Sickle cell	0	1	2	3	4
Other[1]	0	1	2	3	4
E. Personal habits					
Smoking	0	1	2	3	4
Alcohol	0	1	2	3	4
Drugs (marijuana, opiates)	0	1	2	3	4
Caffeine (e.g., cola drinks, coffee)	0	1	2	3	4
Other[1]	0	1	2	3	4

[1] Expand to fit circumstances of particular country or region.

HISTORY OF PREVIOUS PREGNANCIES
(complete one for each pregnancy)

Name of patient _____   Date:_____
Name of trainee _____   *Rating scale*
Name of evaluator _____   0 = Omitted or forgot to develop question
Program _____   1 = Basic technique needs review; question poorly
Site _____   phrased
                                                    2 = Understands basic technique, but needs more
                                                        practice
                                                    3 = Speed, style, and manner good
                                                    4 = Speed, style, and manner excellent

				Rating				
1. Year				0	1	2	3	4
2. Abortion miscarriage								
When? Trimester	1	2	3	0	1	2	3	4
Medical intervention		Y	N	0	1	2	3	4
Elective or spontaneous?		E	S	0	1	2	3	4
3. Complications during pregnancy								
(a) High blood pressure				0	1	2	3	4
(b) Vaginal bleeding				0	1	2	3	4
(c) Infection (e.g., rubella, viral)				0	1	2	3	4
(d) Other[1]				0	1	2	3	4
4. Delivery								
(a) Site				0	1	2	3	4
(b) Hours in labor				0	1	2	3	4
(c) Type of delivery (vaginal, Cesarean)				0	1	2	3	4
(d) Anesthetic				0	1	2	3	4
(e) Maternal complications				0	1	2	3	4
5. Baby								
(a) Sex				0	1	2	3	4
(b) Weight				0	1	2	3	4
(c) Estimated weeks of gestation				0	1	2	3	4
(d) Neonatal complications				0	1	2	3	4
(e) Fed breast or bottle				0	1	2	3	4
(f) Child's present age				0	1	2	3	4
(g) Present health of child				0	1	2	3	4
(h) Problems:								
Anemia				0	1	2	3	4
Allergy				0	1	2	3	4
Infections				0	1	2	3	4
Deficiency diseases				0	1	2	3	4
Other[1]				0	1	2	3	4

[1] Expand to fit circumstances of particular country or region.

Measuring blood pressure

Two components are assessed in evaluating the performance of a student learning to take blood pressure readings: process and outcome.

1. Process: Direct observation of technique and patient interaction
The skilled art of taking blood pressure has been divided into a number of components on the rating form. Some of the components (for example, number 7) are further subdivided. Each component or sub-component is assessed on a 5-point scale in terms of increasing degrees of smoothness and mastery.

If a step is omitted, score 0.
If the basic technique needs review, score 1.
If more practice is needed, score 2.
If technique is *adequate* for working with patients, score 3.
If technique is smooth and very skilled, score 4.

In short, a score of 3 represents minimal mastery (adequate for patient care) and one of 4 denotes a higher level of achievement.

2. Outcome: Blood pressure reading
Auditory confirmation of the blood pressure recorded by the student can be made by an observer taking a reading and comparing it with that taken by the student.

EVALUATION OF BLOOD PRESSURE MEASUREMENT FOR PRENATAL HEALTH CARE BY MATERNAL AND CHILD HEALTH TRAINEE

Name of patient _____   Date_____
Name of trainee _____   *Rating scale*
Name of evaluator _____   0 = This step was omitted
Program_____   1 = The basic technique of this step needs to be reviewed
Site _____   with the student
2 = The student understands the basic technique, but needs more practice
3 = Speed, style, and technique are *adequate* for working with patients
4 = Speed, style, and technique excellent

I. Direct observation

Component tasks		Rating			
1. Explains to the patient what will be done (e.g., "This will feel tight on your arm, but it won't hurt."). Asks, "Have you ever had your blood pressure taken?"	0	1	2	3	4
2. Explains blood pressure in language patient can understand.	0	1	2	3	4
3. Checks size of the blood pressure cuff.					
(a) Holds width of cuff against diameter of arm.	0	1	2	3	4
(b) Selects a cuff of appropriate size, approximately 20 % greater than arm diameter.[1]	0	1	2	3	4
4. Rolls up sleeve of patient's garment so no material will be under cuff.	0	1	2	3	4
5. Centers cuff bladder over the brachial artery.	0	1	2	3	4
6. Positions and supports the arm at heart level.	0	1	2	3	4
7. Takes a palpatory pulse.[2]					
(a) Palpates radial or brachial artery.	0	1	2	3	4
(b) Inflates cuff until arterial pulse can no longer be felt.	0	1	2	3	4
(c) Inflates cuff 1.33 kPa (10 mmHg) higher.	0	1	2	3	4
(d) Deflates cuff at a rate no more than 0.4 kPa·(3 mmHg) sec.	0	1	2	3	4
(e) Records kPa where arterial pulse is again palpated.	0	1	2	3	4
(f) Deflates cuff completely.	0	1	2	3	4
8. Waits 30 seconds, allowing arm to rest (could take heart rate during this time).	0	1	2	3	3
9. Repositions arm at heart level.	0	1	2	3	4
10. Places diaphragm of stethoscope over brachial artery.	0	1	2	3	4
11. Inflates cuff to 2.67 kPa (20 mmHg) above palpatory pulse.	0	1	2	3	4
12. Records auscultatory blood pressure					
(a) Records kPa where first sound heard.	0	1	2	3	4
(b) Records kPa where sounds muffle.	0	1	2	3	4
(c) Records kPa where sounds disappear.	0	1	2	3	4
13. Replaces arm at rest.	0	1	2	3	4
14. Offers patient an opportunity to ask questions.	0	1	2	3	4

II. Auditory confirmation

Student's reading _____

Evaluator's reading_____

Difference_____

Clinically significant   Y   N   ?

[1] If the cuff selected is too large, the blood pressure recorded will be erroneously low. If the cuff is too small, the reading will be erroneously high. Written short-answer or multiple-choice questions can be used to evaluate knowledge of this aspect.
[2] Used to obtain systolic estimate to avoid error from possible auscultatory gap.

Part II

EXAMPLES OF ASSESSMENT INSTRUMENTS

EXPLANATORY NOTE

In this part, a number of instruments used in the performance assessment of students and health workers in several countries are presented. They have been kindly made available by their authors and provide useful examples of the techniques described in Part I.

Many of them are still being worked on. They are therefore not to be viewed as instruments which can or should be applied. Rather, they serve to illustrate techniques. It is hoped that their presentation here will serve to stimulate further development and hence improve performance assessment.

The presentation of instruments is not intended to be comprehensive, i.e., to cover most functions or tasks of health workers. Nor is it confined to instruments that have been systematically evaluated. Few of them meet this criterion. Rather, they serve to illustrate different techniques.

It is intended to update this presentation regularly and it is hoped that readers will provide information to WHO so that new techniques and instruments will be made available for inclusion in future publications.

The instruments have been developed to assess the performance of many different categories of health worker or student: nurses; medical assistants (physician's assistants); laboratory technicians; physical therapists; physicians, etc. However, they are not presented by category of health worker, but classified in three sections as follows:

Section 1. Instruments used to assess the performance of essential task elements of most health care action, e.g., data-gathering, effective interaction with other persons, etc.

Section 2. Instruments used in comprehensive assessments of job performance, i.e., designed to cover the whole range of abilities required to carry out the main functions of a specified category of health worker.

Section 3. Instruments to assess the performance of more specific tasks or components of tasks.

Most of the instruments are in the form of check-lists and rating scales. There are, however, examples of techniques using patient management problems or patient simulation, and of questioning of students (oral examinations).

There are few examples of procedures using the more traditional techniques (essay, short-answer tests, multiple-choice questions), though these undoubtedly might form part of a comprehensive assessment of performance.

Some of the instruments are complex, others relatively simple. All of them, however, will need to be used by personnel specially trained to make judgements, observe accurately, etc. Also it cannot be stressed enough that every instrument will need adaptation to ensure its relevance and appropriateness to local conditions.

To assist the reader, each instrument is preceded by a brief explanatory note. In this the following information is presented:

I. Type of instrument, health care activity involved, and the category of student or health worker for which the instrument was designed or is being used
II. Competences to be assessed
III. Specific abilities to be assessed
IV. Purpose of assessment for which the instrument was developed, including whether it was designed for summative or formative purposes
V. Comments (including information on any systematic evaluation that has been carried out and on any special features of the instrument)
VI. Source, i.e., the name and address of the originator(s) of the instrument for readers wishing to have further information.

Finally, it must be stressed again that the main purpose of this collection of instruments is to stimulate the much needed development of performance assessment techniques. The instruments presented here, by exemplifying what has been done by a few, will—it is hoped—lead to action by many others and will ensure that in the future a whole range of assessment instruments will be at the disposal of teachers and supervisors of health workers.

CLINICAL PROFICIENCY (GENERAL)

Type of instrument	Performance	Category of health personnel	Reference number	Page
Rating scale	Comprehensive clinical proficiency	Medical technologist	1	54
Rating scale	Comprehensive clinical proficiency	Physician's assistant	2	57
Rating scale	Comprehensive clinical proficiency	Physician	3	59
Rating scale	Comprehensive clinical proficiency	Physician – postgraduate	4	63
Patient management problem	Comprehensive clinical proficiency	Physician's assistant	5	66
Rating scale	Comprehensive nursing proficiency	Nurse	6	69
Rating scale	Comprehensive clinical proficiency	Physician	7	73
Rating Scale	Comprehensive clinical proficiency	Physician	8	76

ASSESSMENT INSTRUMENT 1

I. Rating scale: Comprehensive clinical proficiency (medical technologist)

II. Competences to be assessed:
Communication
Interpersonal relations
Problem-solving

III. Specific abilities to be assessed:
1. Ability to execute tests and procedures with efficiency, accuracy, and safety.
2. Ability to organize equipment.
3. Ability to work and communicate easily with patients and colleagues.
4. Ability to record test results neatly and legibly.

IV. Purpose of assessment: summative.
Used as final examination to assess professional competence of medical technologists.

V. Comments:
No evaluation studies reported.

VI. Source to contact for further information:
Mary A. Feeley
Department of Medical Technology
Indiana University—Purdue University
Indianapolis, IN
USA

PROFESSIONAL COMPETENCE

Name_____ Section_____ Evaluator_____

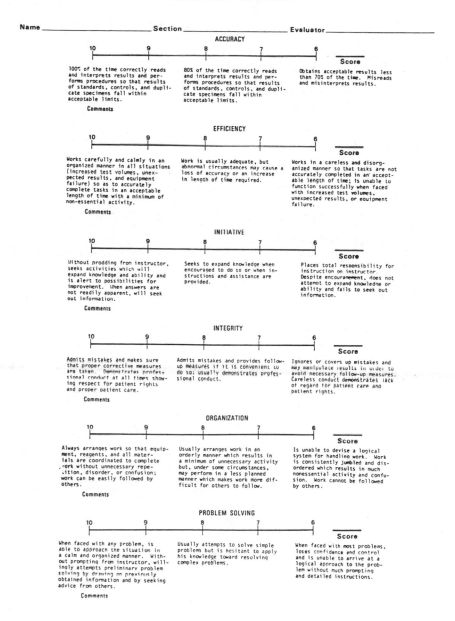

ACCURACY

10	9	8	7	6

Score

100% of the time correctly reads and interprets results and performs procedures so that results of standards, controls, and duplicate specimens fall within acceptable limits.

Comments

80% of the time correctly reads and interprets results and performs procedures so that results of standards, controls, and duplicate specimens fall within acceptable limits.

Obtains acceptable results less than 70% of the time. Misreads and misinterprets results.

EFFICIENCY

10	9	8	7	6

Score

Works carefully and calmly in an organized manner in all situations (increased test volumes, unexpected results, and equipment failure) so as to accurately complete tasks in an acceptable length of time with a minimum of non-essential activity.

Comments

Work is usually adequate, but abnormal circumstances may cause a loss of accuracy or an increase in length of time required.

Works in a careless and disorganized manner so that tasks are not accurately completed in an acceptable length of time; is unable to function successfully when faced with increased test volumes, unexpected results, or equipment failure.

INITIATIVE

10	9	8	7	6

Score

Without prodding from instructor, seeks activities which will expand knowledge and ability and is alert to possibilities for improvement. When answers are not readily apparent, will seek out information.

Comments

Seeks to expand knowledge when encouraged to do so or when instructions and assistance are provided.

Places total responsibility for instruction on instructor. Despite encouragement, does not attempt to expand knowledge or ability and fails to seek out information.

INTEGRITY

10	9	8	7	6

Score

Admits mistakes and makes sure that proper corrective measures are taken. Demonstrates professional conduct at all times showing respect for patient rights and proper patient care.

Comments

Admits mistakes and provides follow-up measures if it is convenient to do so; usually demonstrates professional conduct.

Ignores or covers up mistakes and to avoid necessary follow-up measures. Careless conduct demonstrates lack of regard for patient care and patient rights.

ORGANIZATION

10	9	8	7	6

Score

Always arranges work so that equipment, reagents, and all materials are coordinated to complete work without unnecessary repetition, disorder, or confusion; work can be easily followed by others.

Comments

Usually arranges work in an orderly manner which results in a minimum of unnecessary activity but, under some circumstances, may perform in a less planned manner which makes work more difficult for others to follow.

Is unable to devise a logical system for handling work. Work is consistently jumbled and disordered which results in much nonessential activity and confusion. Work cannot be followed by others.

PROBLEM SOLVING

10	9	8	7	6

Score

When faced with any problem, is able to approach the situation in a calm and organized manner. Without prompting from instructor, willingly attempts preliminary problem solving by drawing on previously obtained information and by seeking advice from others.

Comments

Usually attempts to solve simple problems but is hesitant to apply his knowledge toward resolving complex problems.

When faced with most problems, loses confidence and control and is unable to arrive at a logical approach to the problem without much prompting and detailed instructions.

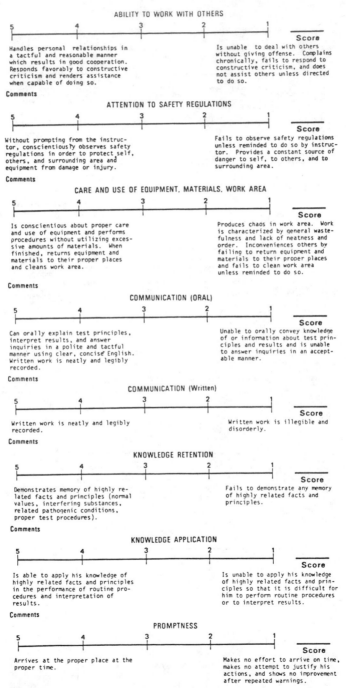

ABILITY TO WORK WITH OTHERS

5   4   3   2   1

Score _____

Handles personal relationships in a tactful and reasonable manner which results in good cooperation. Responds favorably to constructive criticism and renders assistance when capable of doing so.

Is unable to deal with others without giving offense. Complains chronically, fails to respond to constructive criticism, and does not assist others unless directed to do so.

Comments

ATTENTION TO SAFETY REGULATIONS

5   4   3   2   1

Score _____

Without prompting from the instructor, conscientiously observes safety regulations in order to protect self, others, and surrounding area and equipment from damage or injury.

Fails to observe safety regulations unless reminded to do so by instructor. Provides a constant source of danger to self, to others, and to surrounding area.

Comments

CARE AND USE OF EQUIPMENT, MATERIALS, WORK AREA

5   4   3   2   1

Score _____

Is conscientious about proper care and use of equipment and performs procedures without utilizing excessive amounts of materials. When finished, returns equipment and materials to their proper places and cleans work area.

Produces chaos in work area. Work is characterized by general wastefulness and lack of neatness and order. Inconveniences others by failing to return equipment and materials to their proper places and fails to clean work area unless reminded to do so.

Comments

COMMUNICATION (ORAL)

5   4   3   2   1

Score _____

Can orally explain test principles, interpret results, and answer inquiries in a polite and tactful manner using clear, concise English. Written work is neatly and legibly recorded.

Unable to orally convey knowledge of or information about test principles and results and is unable to answer inquiries in an acceptable manner.

Comments

COMMUNICATION (Written)

5   4   3   2   1

Score _____

Written work is neatly and legibly recorded.

Written work is illegible and disorderly.

Comments

KNOWLEDGE RETENTION

5   4   3   2   1

Score _____

Demonstrates memory of highly related facts and principles (normal values, interfering substances, related pathogenic conditions, proper test procedures).

Fails to demonstrate any memory of highly related facts and principles.

Comments

KNOWLEDGE APPLICATION

5   4   3   2   1

Score _____

Is able to apply his knowledge of highly related facts and principles in the performance of routine procedures and interpretation of results.

Is unable to apply his knowledge of highly related facts and principles so that it is difficult for him to perform routine procedures or to interpret results.

Comments

PROMPTNESS

5   4   3   2   1

Score _____

Arrives at the proper place at the proper time.

Makes no effort to arrive on time, makes no attempt to justify his actions, and shows no improvement after repeated warnings.

Comments

ASSESSMENT INSTRUMENT 2

I. Rating scale: Comprehensive clinical proficiency (physician's assistant)

II. Competences to be assessed:
Data-gathering
Data interpretation
Communication
Reporting

III. Specific abilities to be assessed:
1. Ability to identify patient's problem accurately.
2. Ability to perform diagnostic and therapeutic procedures.
3. Ability to identify, for referral, cases beyond own level of competence.
4. Ability to use and maintain medical records.
5. Ability to work cooperatively with patients and their families as well as with staff.
6. Ability to organize and carry out assignments responsibly and effectively.

IV. Purpose of assessment: summative.
Designed to be used on completion of training of physician's assistants to assess overall clinical competence.

V. Comments:
Instrument is currently in use in physician's assistant training programme. No formal evaluation or statistical data are available.

VI. Source to contact for further information:
Rosemarie Yidela
Physician's Assistant Program Director
United States Public Health Service Hospital
Staten Island, NY 10304
USA

PHYSICIAN'S ASSISTANT TRAINING PROGRAM
STUDENT CLINICAL EVALUATION

Student _____

Service assignment _____

Dates of assignment _____

Dear Doctor _____

Please use the following number code when evaluating this student's level of ability:

Excellent = 4; Good = 3; Average = 2; Unsatisfactory = 1

Code

1. Elicits an accurate and complete patient history.
2. Performs an accurate and complete physical examination.
3. Accurately identifies the patient's problem.
4. Determines action(s) appropriate to the patient's problem, including referral to a physician.
5. Ability to perform diagnostic and therapeutic procedures.
6. Demonstrates knowledge of applicable medical, biological, and physical sciences.
7. Utilizes and accurately maintains medical records, as allowed.
8. Recognizes own limitations.
9. Exhibits ethical behavior and attitudes.
10. Maintains professional relations with staff.
11. Maintains professional relations with patient and family.
12. Communicates ideas and information effectively.
13. Plans, organizes, and carries out responsibilities effectively.
14. Dress and appearance.
15. Attendance and punctuality.
16. Acceptance of constructive criticism.

Preceptors are urged to discuss the student's performance and evaluation with them. Please have the student comment on and sign this form before returning it to this program.

Preceptor's comments:

_____

Date   Student's signature

_____

Date   Preceptor's signature and title

Student's comments:

ASSESSMENT INSTRUMENT 3

I. Rating scale: Comprehensive clinical proficiency (physician)

II. Competences to be assessed:
Data-gathering
Problem-solving
Planning patient management

III. Specific abilities to be assessed:
1. Ability to obtain essential medical and social history in a sensitive professional manner.
2. Ability to record pertinent information briefly but thoroughly.
3. Ability to organize, interpret, and communicate clinical findings.
4. Ability to select best alternatives among diagnoses and plans for treatment.

IV. Purpose of assessment: formative.
Intended for periodic use, during a medical course, for rating patient workups.

V. Comments:
The rating form is an adaptation of the Arizona Clinical Interview Rating Scale.[1] No systematic studies available relative to reliability. Provides clear descriptions of behaviour at advanced, acceptable, and unacceptable levels with relation to general but specified areas of competence.

VI. Source to contact for further information:
Andrea K. Schroder
Instructor
Departments of Preventive Medicine and Psychiatry
University of Colorado Medical Center
Denver, CO 80262
USA

---

[1] STILLMAN, P. L. ET AL. *Pediatrics*, 57: 769–774 (1976).

CLINICAL SKILL ASSESSMENT SCALE

Points   *Criteria*

I. Rapport

Explores concerns

5   The interviewer seemed alert, sensitive, and responsive to the patient and to possible concerns expressed by the patient regardless of whether such concerns were immediately relevant to the area being discussed; e.g., marital problems, child discipline problems, depression. Interviewer was able to explore concerns in sufficient depth.

4

3   The interviewer was responsive to the patient and able to detect concerns expressed by the patient, but failed to explore them in sufficient depth.

2

1   The interviewer seemed indifferent and was unalert and/or insensitive to possible concerns expressed by the patient. For whatever reason the interviewer tended to avoid discussing possible problem areas which could have either immediate or future implications for the mental or physical health of his patient.

Posture, deportment, dress

5   The interviewer's posture, deportment, and dress reflected a sense of professionalism and maturity appropriate to the doctor-patient relationship.

4

3   The interviewer was adequate in his/her posture, deportment, dress.

2

1   The interviewer's posture, deportment, and dress were substandard for his/her role. He/she failed in this area to display adequate professionalism and maturity appropriate to the doctor-patient relationship.

II. Organization

Covers major areas

5   The interviewer progresses through the major subsections of the medical history in proper sequence.

4

3   The interviewer covers all of the major subsections of the history but in the wrong sequence.

2

1   The interviewer omits major subsections of the history.

Directs interview

5   The interviewer formally directs the interview so that the main purpose is achieved. When necessary, interviewer actively intervenes with tact and appropriate timing rather than "railroading" the patient away from his concerns and priorities.

4

3   The interviewer generally directs the interview but has difficulty maintaining the focus and/or intervening appropriately with more difficult patients.

2

1   The interviewer does not formally direct the interview or attempt to maintain a purposeful focus during the interview.

III. Review of systems

5   Asks the right questions and is attentive to the answers. Follows up vague replies with appropriate questions.

4

3   Asks the right questions, but often in a mechanical way. Rarely misses important information, but tends to follow it up only superficially.

2

1   Omits important questions. Does not follow up important information that he/she does elicit. Is inattentive and often fails to listen carefully to answers. Frequently fails to use information from the review of systems in formulating and analysing the patient's problems.

IV. Written material

Brevity, pertinence

5   Case write-ups are brief, yet important and pertinent data are not omitted.

4

3   Case write-ups are acceptable, however brevity/pertinence (circle one or both) need(s) improvement.

2

1   Case write-ups are awkward. Sentence structure is unwieldy. Student fails to extrapolate important data.

V. Verbal presentations

5   Concise, well-organized. Gives clear picture of patients and their problems. Shows poise. Accepts criticism well and makes use of it.

4

V. Verbal presentations (contd.)

3   Somewhat longer than necessary, but well organized and informative. Somewhat ill at ease and mechanical in his/her presentation, but responds well to questions and criticism.

2
1   Rambling, disorganized presentations. Student excessively nervous. Thinks poorly when asked questions in the course of the presentation. Resentful of criticism.

VI. Clinical reasoning and judgement

Ability to identify problems

5   Defines problems accurately and shows good judgement in determining their order of importance. Problem lists are complete, with appropriate emphasis on each problem.

4
3   Defines the most important problems, but lacks consistency in assigning them appropriate priorities. Problem lists sometimes incomplete, but rarely omits major problems.

2
1   Frequently omits major problems. Problems are poorly defined, indicating a poor understanding of the clinical information. Poor sense of priority in his/her approach to multiple problems.

Ability to organize, distil, and analyse clinical data

5   Is meticulous and accurate in assembling clinical information and condensing it. Organizes the information clearly and concisely, and has a good sense of how to relate the information to the patient's problems.

4
3   Assembles clinical information accurately and thoroughly. Inconsistent in his/her ability to relate clinical information to the patient's problems.

2
1   Clinical information is frequently inaccurate or incomplete. Fails to organize facts in a logical way. Frequently reaches conclusions that are not based on available information.

Ability to formulate working hypotheses based on clinical data

5   Shows sound reasoning in drawing conclusions from available clinical data. When he/she does speculate, he/she is aware of it and says so. Shows appropriate scepticism toward his /her working hypothesis and a willingness to change it as additional data dictate.

4
3   Shows sound reasoning in drawing conclusions from additional data, but tends to state conclusions without indicating how he/she arrived at them. Seldom reaches conclusions that are not justified by the data. Is usually willing to change his/her interpretation if new data warrant it.

2
1   Often confused about the meaning of clinical information and draws illogical conclusions from it. Does not distinguish well between conclusions based on available information and conclusions based on speculation. Adheres too rigidly to his/her conclusions even when available evidence shows them to be wrong.

Ability to make plans for diagnosis, treatment, and patient education

5   Plans are thoroughly considered and appropriate.
4
3   Always puts forward plans and they are usually appropriate. However, they are often sketchy and poorly defined.

2
1   Often fails to put a plan forward. When he/she does, it is poorly organized and frequently irrelevant to the patient's problems.

Ability to consider logical alternatives

5   Gives thorough consideration to alternative interpretations to those he/she puts forward. The alternatives are realistic explanations for the particular problem at hand. Is appropriately flexible in altering his/her conclusions in light of new information, but is not easily swayed by inconclusive data or by the opinions and speculation of others.

4
3   Consistently arrives at logical conclusions, but keeps an open mind about logical alternatives. Usually considers the most likely alternatives, rarely suggests impossible ones, but does tend to omit uncommon possibilities.

2
1   Prone to develop "tunnel vision" about a problem and often fails to acknowledge possible explanations other than the one he/she favors. Adheres rigidly to his/her conclusions even in the light of information which shows them to be wrong. Shows little interest in alternative solutions to a problem.

Date: _____ Student: _____

	Advanced	Acceptable		Unacceptable
I. Rapport				
A. Explores concerns	5	4	3	2	1
B. Posture, deportment, dress	5	4	3	2	1
II. Organization				
A. Covers major areas	5	4	3	2	1
B. Directs interview	5	4	3	2	1
III. Review of systems	5	4	3	2	1
IV. Written material				
A. Brevity, pertinence	5	4	3	2	1
V. Verbal presentations	5	4	3	2	1
VI. Clinical reasoning and judgement				
A. Ability to identify problems	5	4	3	2	1
B. Ability to organize and analyse clinical data	5	4	3	2	1
C. Ability to formulate working hypotheses based on clinical data	5	4	3	2	1
D. Ability to make plans	5	4	3	2	1
E. Ability to consider logical alternatives	5	4	3	2	1

ASSESSMENT INSTRUMENT 4

I. Rating scale: Comprehensive clinical proficiency (physician—postgraduate)

II. Competences to be assessed:
Data-gathering
Recording
Interpreting
Communicating
Planning patient care

III. Specific abilities to be assessed:
1. Ability to take comprehensive history and perform accurate physical examination.
2. Ability to report cases clearly and accurately.
3. Ability to manage patient care constructively and independently.
4. Ability to work smoothly and effectively in interpersonal relationships.
5. Ability to apply scientific data to the solution of health problems.

IV. Purpose of assessment: summative.
Used in rotation programme to assess overall clinical competence at the end of each service—medical postgraduate (interns, residents, fellows).

V. Comments:
Instrument has been evaluated and statistical data are available on reliability, as well as predictive analysis studies. Has useful discussion of common rating errors to be avoided.

VI. Source to contact for further information:
Dr Richard S. Gallagher
Director
Division of Educational Service and Research
School of Medicine
Wayne State University
540 East Canfield
Detroit, MI 48202
USA

POSTGRADUATE TRAINEE RATING FORM
FORM H
INSTRUCTIONS

PLEASE READ THESE INSTRUCTIONS BEFORE COMPLETING THE RATING FORM:

On this form you will find a number of traits which have been identified as describing characteristics of professional trainees (interns, residents, and fellows) which are important components of professional competence.

Each of these traits is to be rated on a continuum which has two opposite poles with different "degrees" of the trait in between poles. Along the continuum are short descriptive phrases (anchors) which describe different degrees or amounts of a particular trait. These phrases are simple guideposts.

To record your rating, simply *check* (√) the line at the point which in your best judgment describes the professional trainee on a particular trait. Your ratings can fall at the anchor or anywhere between anchors. In general, the finer your discrimination of a trainee's performance on a particular trait, the more accurate your rating will be.

Your rating should reflect the trainee's performance with respect to the standard for his group and training level and in accord with the anchors which describe performance.

If you feel that you have not had sufficient opportunity to evaluate a trainee on a particular trait, indicate "NOT OBSERVED" by placing a check (√) in the box adjacent to the trait.

CAUTION!

The following are common rating errors which will tend to make your ratings less reliable. Please be conscious of your own tendency to make these errors as you complete the ratings. Be as precise and objective as possible.

COMMON RATING ERRORS:

1. Error of Leniency. Raters tend to rate those whom they know well or like *higher* than they should.

2. Error of Central Tendency. Raters hesitate to give extreme judgments and thus tend to displace very high or very low ratings in the direction of the mean of a group.

3. Halo effect. Raters tend to make judgments on one trait on the basis of their feelings about other characteristics of the trainee. For example, your feelings about a trainee's appearance may color your views of his diagnostic ability.

4. Logical Error. Raters tend to give similar ratings for traits that seem logically related in the mind of the rater. For example, there may be a tendency to give similar ratings on diagnostic ability and oral verbal ability when this is not justified.

5. Proximity Error. Raters tend to give similar ratings on traits which are adjacent to one another in the rating form.

6. Contrast Error. Raters tend to rate individuals in the opposite direction from the rater's perception of his own ability on a given trait. For example, if a rater sees himself as having an extremely high level of intellectual curiosity, he will tend to rate others lower on this trait than most other raters.

☐ INTERN
☐ RESIDENT
☐ FELLOW　NAME:_____

RATER:_____　　RATER'S POSITION:_____
TYPE OF ROTATION:_____　　HOSPITAL:_____
PERIOD FROM: __/__/__ TO: __/__/__　　SIGNATURE:_____

HISTORY TAKING

Obtains history which is often incomplete and/or inaccurate; has difficulty with organization. | Able to obtain thorough history but does not always pursue other sources when indicated and occasionally will have important omissions. Generally well organized. | Uniformly able to elicit a comprehensive history from patients; consistently uses sources other than the patient to supplement history when indicated and organizes data well.

☐ Not Observed

PHYSICAL EXAM

Physical examinations usually have minor and may also have major deficiencies in technical quality and thoroughness. | Usually performs precise and complete examination, but may have minor deficiencies on occasion. | Always performs a technically accurate and complete physical examination.

☐ Not Observed

CASE PRESENTATION

Frequently uses incorrect terminology, uncertain of precise meanings, is difficult to follow. | Uses correct terminology but most of the time is disorganized and unable to communicate thoughts to others. | Usually clear, but occasionally disorganized and unable to communicate thoughts to others. | Easy to follow; gives accurate presentation of the most pressing problems; tends to overlook less urgent but nevertheless important problems. | Easy to follow; routinely accurate presentations of all problems and the patient's progress.

☐ Not Observed

RECORD-KEEPING ABILITY

Frequently has incomplete records, patient's problems and progress are not easily identifiable. | Routinely writes legible, clear, and accurate reports but tends to overlook problems and indicators of progress which appear less urgent. | Routinely has legible, clear, up-to-date, and accurate records. Patient's problems and progress are easily identifiable.

☐ Not Observed

CLINICAL JUDGMENT & DIAGNOSTIC ABILITY

Clincial rationale is commonly haphazard even with simple problems. Routinely uses diagnostic procedures inefficiently and ineffectively. | Demonstrates occasional deficiencies with simple as well as complex problems. Occasionally misinterprets, misjudges clinical information. | Consistently makes carefully reasoned deductions from history and physical examination; rationale for selecting laboratory procedures is always mature and well founded.

☐ Not Observed

PATIENT MANAGEMENT

Common problems are sometimes managed poorly; rarely if ever contributes constructive new perceptions to difficult problems. | Handles most common clinical problems satisfactorily; occasionally pursues a well-reasoned, independent approach to difficult problems. | Consistently has a creative, constructive and self-reliant approach to management of difficult as well as common problems. Frequently contributes new insights to problems.

☐ Not Observed

PHYSICIAN-PATIENT RELATIONSHIPS

Often antagonizes or generates a negative reaction from patients. | Patient relationships are superficial; rarely if ever establishes effective rapport. | Relates well to those patients considered "interesting"; tends to ignore others. | Able to relate effectively to most patients, but has yet to learn how to handle difficult situations. | Able to establish effective rapport with all types of patients. Wins the confidence and co-operation of all.

☐ Not Observed

COOPERATION WITH PERSONNEL

Actions are often thoughtless and cause unnecessary work and emotional stress for other personnel. | Generally does own work but neither helps nor hinders the work of others. | Carries full share of responsibility and is always thoughtful and concerned about helping other professional and allied health personnel to do their jobs effectively.

☐ Not Observed

TEACHING ABILITY

Makes no observable nor planned contribution to the learning process of others. | On occasion helps others to learn, but provides little stimulus for learning by others. | Makes overt efforts to help others learn on regular basis and is usually an effective teacher. | Consistently is an effective and stimulating teacher both in the way tasks are assigned and organized and through verbal communication.

☐ Not Observed

KNOWLEDGE BASE

Unsatisfactory. | Doubtful. | Satisfactory. | Good. | Outstanding.

☐ Not Observed

OVERALL CLINICAL COMPETENCE

Unsatisfactory. | Doubtful. | Satisfactory. | Good. | Outstanding.

☐ Not Observed

FORM 10-1110 2.5M 10-76

ASSESSMENT INSTRUMENT 5

I. Patient management problem: Comprehensive clinical proficiency (physician's assistant)

II. Competences to be assessed:
Data-gathering
Diagnosis
Case management

III. Specific abilities to be assessed:
1. Ability to obtain relevant patient history and symptoms.
2. Ability to select appropriate laboratory tests and procedures.
3. Ability to interpret data correctly for purposes of diagnosis.

IV. Purpose of assessment: summative.
As comprehensive examination at end of sequence of courses for physician's assistant.

V. Comments:
Instrument has not been evaluated and no specific validity data are available. In current use.

VI. Source to contact for further information:
Physician Assistant Program
The George Washington University Medical Center
Washington, DC
USA

CASE PROBLEM

(Page 1)

Mary Ellen E. is a twelve-year-old student who comes to the physician's office because of a persistent sore throat. About a week ago she began having a sore throat, mild fever and chills, headache, fatigue, and general malaise. The fever, which she didn't measure, seems to have subsided for the most part, as has the headache, but the sore throat and the fatigue have continued without improvement. Her sleep has been restless and her appetite poor.

1. At this point, what additional questions would you like to ask on history?

_ any respiratory symptoms: cough, cold, runny nose, sputum production
_ any gastrointestinal symptoms: nausea, vomiting, diarrhea
_ any past history of sore throat, "strep" throat, rheumatic fever, mononucleosis
_ any other significant past medical history, medication, immunization history
_ questions to define "fatigue"—how much, relation to activities, any history of anemia
_ aggravating or relieving factors, treatments tried, effect of illness upon patient
_ known exposure to others with similar symptoms: are any other family members ill?

(Possible points: 7)

(Student gives in page 1 before getting page 2.)

(Page 2)

On further questioning you learn that she has no other noticeable symptoms, no significant past or present medical problems, and no known exposure to others with similar symptoms. No one else in the family is ill. She has been staying home from school and has been too tired to do much more than watch TV. Immunizations are complete.

On physical exam you find the following:

T — 101.2 F.   P — 84, reg.   BP — 116/78

General: The patient is a slightly overweight white female; no acute distress.

Skin: Few acneiform lesions on the face. Also questionable faint maculopapular rash on chest and upper extremities.

EENT: Eyes, ears, nose—within normal limits. No nasal discharge. Oropharynx is markedly injected with low-grade lymphoid hyperplasia; tonsils are 2 + in size, hyperemic, and have a grayish exudate bilaterally.

Neck: Moderately enlarged, tender cervical adenopathy bilaterally involving the anterior and posterior triangles. Thyroid not enlarged.

Chest: Clear to percussion and auscultation. Bilateral fine axillary adenopathy, non-tender.

Heart: Grade II/VI systolic ejection murmur at apex radiating to axilla. (Patient tells you she has been told by other physicians about this.)

Abdomen: Liver 6 cm by percussion, edge palpable and slightly tender at costal margin. Spleen palpable 3 cm below costal margin and is moderately tender. No abdominal distention or masses. Normal bowel sounds. Bilateral inguinal adenopathy—firm, small, non-tender.

Extremities: Within normal limits.

2. What is your differential diagnosis at this point?

1 point each for: mononucleosis, streptococcal pharyngitis, viral pharyngitis, acute leukemia.
1 extra credit point for cytomegalovirus mononucleosis.
No points, but not wrong for: diphtheria, rubella, hepatitis, rheumatic fever, juvenile rheumatoid arthritis.

(Possible points: 4)

3. What laboratory tests would you want to order?

1 point each for: complete blood count (CBC) or white blood cells (WBC), throat culture, heterophil antibody test (or Monospot).
No credit but not wrong for liver function studies.
Epstein-Barr virus-specific serodiagnostic test is wrong answer here (too expensive and not necessary).

(Possible points: 3)

(Give in page 2 before getting page 3.)

(Page 3)

You order a throat culture, CBC, liver function studies, and heterophil antibody test. In one hour you have the following results:

(1) Hemoglobin (Hgb)—13.2 g/100 ml Hematocrit (Hct)—40%
    WBC—13 000   30% neutrophils, 3% eosinophils, 1% basophils, 10% monocytes, 56% lymphocytes. Approx. 15% of the lymphocytes are atypical forms.
(2) Heterophil antibody test—weakly positive.

3. What is your diagnosis at this point?
(Correct answer: Infectious mononucleosis)

(5 points)

4. What would you do now?
   (a) hospitalize the patient for workup,
   (b) reassure patient that her disease is benign and send her home for rest and observation, or
   (c) give antibiotics and await results of throat culture.

   (Correct answer: (b))

(2 points)

(Give in page 3 before getting page 4)

(Page 4)
The next day you get the following reports:
   Throat culture negative at 24 hours.
   SGOT—75 units/ml (normal 5–40)
   SGPT—60 units/ml (normal 5–35)
   Alk. phos.—6.2 Bodansky units (normal 2.0–4.5)
   bilirubin (total)—1.4 mg% (normal 0.2–0.9)

5. Would you change your previous diagnosis or management in the light of these results? If so, explain why.
   (Correct answer: No)

(2 points)

(Give in page 4 before getting page 5)

(page 5)
You talk to your preceptor, who concurs with your initial impression of infectious mononucleosis. Transient elevations of liver function studies occur in 90% of patients with mononucleosis and will return to normal with recovery.

6. What special precautions, if any, should patients with mononucleosis take?
   (Correct answer: Avoid abdominal trauma (ruptured spleen))

(2 points)

(Total possible points: 25)

ASSESSMENT INSTRUMENT 6

I. Rating scale: Comprehensive nursing proficiency

II. Competences to be assessed:
Data-gathering
Patient care management
Patient education
Communication

III. Specific abilities to be assessed:
1. Ability to base nursing practice on a process of assessment, planning, implementation, and evaluation.
2. Ability to direct and carry out the elements of a patient care programme.
3. Willingness to participate in activities to increase skills and knowledge.
4. Responsibility, as evidenced by pursuit of own professional goals and adherence to institutional policy.
5. Ability to plan, carry out, and evaluate teaching.
6. Ability to exchange information with peers and patients effectively.

IV. Purpose of assessment: formative.
Used to assess general nursing proficiency and to correct problem areas in POR [problem-oriented research] documentation. Used periodically.

V. Comments:
Instrument has been evaluated informally in that it has been used in several clinical areas and results compared.

VI. Source to contact for further information:
Mrs Sandra Merkel
Clinical Nursing Specialist
Mott Children's Hospital
The University of Michigan
Ann Arbor, MI
USA

REGISTERED NURSE PERFORMANCE EVALUATION

Name: ————————————————————————
Class: ————————————————————————
Date: ————————————————————————
Unit: ————————————————————————

1. Nursing practice—the process of assessment, planning, implementation, and evaluation as a basis for practice.

A. Assessment:
  1. Collects pertinent data to identify patient strengths and nursing care problems
     (a) patient interviews
     (b) interviews with family and or other key persons
     (c) medical record
     (d) collaboration with other health team members
     (e) clinical observation and examination
  2. Identifies nursing care problems on the basis of the information collected.

Comments:

B. Planning (participates in developing, or develops, the nursing care plan):

  1. Determines appropriate nursing interventions including preventive nursing measures.
  2. Determines priorities of care.
  3. Writes out the care plan in clear and measurable terms.
  4. Determines that the individual plan of care is consistent with the standard nursing care plan and is congruent with other planned therapies.
  5. Includes discharge plans and goals in the nursing care plan.
  6. Mobilizes equipment and resources necessary for successful implementation of the nursing care plan.
  7. Involves the patient and/or other key persons in planning care when appropriate.

Comments:

C. Implementation:

  1. Demonstrates the clinical skills necessary to carry out the nursing interventions.
  2. Identifies the rationale for nursing interventions.
  3. Sets priorities in delivering patient care.
  4. Elicits participation and cooperation of patient and other key persons in the delivery of care.
  5. Utilizes opportunities to teach health care concepts to the patient and/or other key persons.
  6. Follows up the nursing care plan developed.

Comments:

D. Evaluation:

  1. Routinely evaluates the effects of the nursing care provided.
     (a) Assesses the patient's progress toward health or highest level of functioning.
     (b) Assesses the acceptance by the patient and/or other key persons of the care delivered.
     (c) Assesses the patient's comprehension of the particular health care problem and the care required.
  2. Revises care plan when necessary, utilizing current data.
     (a) Is willing to test new nursing care techniques and methodologies.
     (b) Utilizes information from other health team members.
     (c) Initiates consultation when appropriate.

Comments:

II. Management skills—those organizational skills necessary for the efficient direction and implementation of the appropriate components of a patient care delivery system for a particular unit area.

A. Assessment of organizational needs:
  1. Collects necessary information regarding work tasks and allocated resources.
  2. Anticipates potential work-flow problems.
  3. Identifies available and potential resources.
  4. Identifies actions necessary to accomplish work tasks.
  5. Identifies alternate actions.
  6. Implements appropriate actions.

The right margin of the form contains three vertical rating columns labelled: rarely, frequently, consistently.

B. Direction of others:
1. Directs the activities of designated staff.
2. Sets priorities for the completion of work tasks and delegates responsibilities among available qualified staff.
3. Sees that work tasks are completed.

C. Evaluation of unit operation:
1. Evaluates the performance of designated staff.
2. Takes appropriate action to correct unacceptable practices of designated staff.
3. Contributes to the efficiency of the area/unit, e.g., by offering suggestions for change, improvement in methods of organization or delivery of care, greater flexibility.

Comments:

III. Professional education and self-development—participation in formal and informal learning opportunities to increase skills and knowledge.

A. Attends staff development and in-service programs:
1. Recommended for all unit staff.
2. Other programs.
B. Attends continuing education programs.
C. Reads literature pertaining to area of practice.
D. Plans for own continued learning through participation in a variety of activities.
E. Implements in practice setting knowledge and skills gained (list examples in space below)
F. Participates in activities to share expertise (list examples in space below).

Comments:

IV. Responsibility—adherence to policies and procedures and assumption of initiative for improving personal and institutional practices.

A. Adherence to policies and procedures:
1. Adheres to institutional, departmental, and unit policies and procedures.
2. Identifies improvements in policy and initiates policy changes through appropriate mechanisms.
B. Personal practice:
1. Uses unstructured time constructively.
2. Identifies deficiencies in personal performance; takes action to correct his/her errors; seeks appropriate resources to improve his/her practice.
3. Maintains confidentiality and privacy of recipients of services.
4. Establishes professional goals and pursues and accomplishes them within reasonable time limits.

Comments:

V. Teaching—the process of imparting knowledge to improve comprehension, skills, and sensitivity.

A. Assessment:
1. Assesses the need for information.
2. Assesses the degree and level of information needed.
3. Assesses the level of understanding.
4. Assesses the readiness of the learner to utilize information.

B. Objective formulation:
1. Identifies the goals to be obtained through teaching.
2. Seeks to incorporate the goals of the learner in teaching.
3. Sets realistic goals with the learner.

C. Program planning:
1. Designs teaching plans.
2. Sets realistic time limits for accomplishment.
3. Conveys plans in clear, workable manner and records them appropriately.
4. Contacts appropriate resource personnel for assistance.
5. Plans method of evaluation.

D. Implementation:
1. Follows through with planned program.
2. Conveys information clearly.

rarely frequently consistently

V. Teaching (contd.)

E. Evaluation:
  1. Uses feedback to appraise effectiveness of teaching.
  2. Adjusts plan appropriately to input and feedback.
  3. Adjusts plan as necessary to meet changing needs.

Comments:

	rarely	frequently	consistently

VI. Communication—the process of information exchange.

A. Written:
  1. Maintains patient records which are:
    (*a*) complete and concise,
    (*b*) legible,
    (*c*) completed in a timely fashion.
  2. Maintains non-patient records which are complete, concise, and timely.

B. Verbal:
  1. Communicates with peers in a concise, tactful, and considerate manner.
  2. Communicates with other hospital staff in a concise, tactful, and considerate manner.
  3. Communicates with patients, families, and the public in a concise, tactful, and considerate manner.

C. Interpersonal relations (self-awareness):
  1. Identifies own feelings and attitudes.
  2. Recognizes the effect of personal feelings and attitudes on performance.
  3. Seeks counsel and support from appropriate persons in the event of feelings interfering with performance.

D. Relationships with others:
  1. Listens carefully and objectively to others.
  2. Responds appropriately to constructive suggestions.
  3. Promotes and demonstrates cooperative relationships with hospital staff, patients, and the public.

Comments:

Additional comments:

Supervisor ————Date ————————————
Employee ——————————————————————

ASSESSMENT INSTRUMENT 7

I. Rating scale: Comprehensive clinical proficiency (physician)

II. Competences to be assessed:
Data-gathering
Recording
Interpreting
Planning patient care
Communication

III. Specific abilities to be assessed:
1. Ability to take essential history and perform appropriate physical, social, and mental status examination.
2. Ability to record pertinent patient data in a concise, organized manner.
3. Ability to plan and manage patient care logically and capably.
4. Ability to request and interpret appropriate laboratory procedures.
5. Ability to work responsibly and cooperatively with patient and members of health care team.
6. Ability to identify patient problems that should be referred to a specialist.

IV. Purpose of assessment: summative.
Used at end of a period of service in the training of a medical student, intern, or resident.

V. Comments:
This is a revised version, upon which further research is being done. Instrument has been evaluated and reliability found low.

VI. Source to contact for further information:
Harold G. Levine, Director
Office of Research in Medical Education
University of Texas Medical School
Galveston, TX 77551
USA

CLINICAL PROFICIENCY ASSESSMENT

SECTIONS I - III are not intended to be equated with a grade but represent an assessment of performance in selected areas. The ratings will be used to provide students with feedback.

Instructions: Circle only one response

Circle X if you have inadequate data on which to base judgment
Circle 1 if the student did not or rarely demonstrated the described behavior
Circle 2 if the demonstrated the described behavior with moderate frequency
Circle 3 if the student almost always demonstrated the described behavior

Demonstrated Behavior

INFORMATION GATHERING AND UNDERSTANDING OF MANAGEMENT	Insufficient contact to judge	Rarely or Never	Moderately Often	Almost Always
1 Organizes time efficiently, completes tasks promptly	X	1	2	3
2 Obtains and records appropriate medical history	X	1	2	3
3 Performs and records appropriate physical and/or mental status examination	X	1	2	3
4 Knows when and how to pursue exams beyond screening procedures	X	1	2	3
5 Integrates data obtained from history, physical examination and laboratories into logical formulation of patient's problems	X	1	2	3
6 Is capable of requesting, justifying and interpreting appropriate laboratory examinations or procedures	X	1	2	3
7 Develops logical plan for management, explaining rationale for approach taken	X	1	2	3
8 Identifies socio-economic and ethnic factors which impinge on patient management	X	1	2	3
9 Evaluates and records response to treatment in concise, organized written notes	X	1	2	3
10 Develops appropriate follow-up management plans	X	1	2	3
11 Uses resource materials (books, journals, etc.) to help under stand and solve patient problems	X	1	2	3
12 Is willing to re-examine data base and previous decisions, and to test assessments of problems	X	1	2	3
13 Reacts appropriately to emergency situations, evaluates seriousness and establishes priorities	X	1	2	3
14 Shows initiative in undertaking tasks	X	1	2	3
15 Recognizes his/her professional capabilities and limitations	X	1	2	3

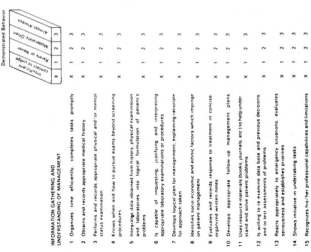

	Insufficient contact to judge	Rarely or Never	Moderately Often	Almost Always
II INTERPERSONAL ABILITIES WITH PATIENTS				
1 Demonstrates consideration, tact and courtesy with patients	X	1	2	3
2 Accepts and encourages expressions of feelings in non judgmental fashion	X	1	2	3
3 Explains procedures (diagnosis and treatment) in effort to relieve patient's discomfort and anxiety	X	1	2	3
4 Establishes a relationship with patient's family, responding to their need for information and using them appropriately in treatment plans	X	1	2	3
5 Gains cooperation and confidence of patients, devotes the time and effort necessary for establishing rapport	X	1	2	3
III INTERPERSONAL ABILITIES WITH OTHER PROFESSIONALS				
1 Recognizes and respects skills of other health care team members, knows how and when to involve them in a treatment plan	X	1	2	3
2 Works cooperatively with and accepts justifiable criticism from those in authority	X	1	2	3
3 Demonstrates an awareness of moral and ethical issues related to medicine through words and actions	X	1	2	3
4 Accepts appropriate share of the students' work responsibilities	X	1	2	3

IV This section will be used to provide a GRADE. Based upon the data from the previous sections, circle the number which indicates the student's overall competence.

If **clear** evidence of inadequacy **was** found that makes **you certain** that the student's performance was inadequate. **clearly failing** or F.   1

If **sufficient** evidence of inadequacy **was found that you would want** the student's performance to be thoroughly investigated before he/she could progress. **probably failing or possible F**   2

If you found some evidence or inadequate performance that might be a problem if others have noticed similar behavior. **marginal or D performance.**   3

If clearly adequate, but much improvement would be desirable. **C performance.**   4

If clearly above adequate, **low B performance**   5

If substantially above adequate. **high B performance.**   6

If superior performance. **A performance.**   7

V Please provide legible COMMENTS about this particular student's knowledge, performance and attitudes

STUDENT'S NAME _____

STUDENT'S I.D. # _____

ROTATION _____

ROTATION DATE _____ to _____

RATER'S NAME _____

THIS EVALUATION IS BASED ON _____ (NUMBER OF)
CONTACTS WITH THE ABOVE NAMED STUDENT.

ASSESSMENT INSTRUMENT 8

I. Rating scale: Comprehensive clinical proficiency (physician)

II. Competences to be assessed:
Data-gathering
Problem-solving
Communication
Treatment-planning

III. Specific abilities assessed:
1. Ability to elicit significant medical, family, and social history.
2. Ability to obtain data needed for differential diagnosis.
3. Ability to plan appropriate therapeutic programme.
4. Skill in employing medical tests and procedures.
5. Ability to record and communicate data briefly but thoroughly.
6. Ability to interact effectively with patients and colleagues.

IV. Purpose of assessment: formative.
Intended for use in periodic review of growth in professional capabilities of medical student.

V. Comments:
Instrument has been evaluated statistically and data are available.

VI. Source to contact for further information.
Ann Davidge
University of Michigan Medical School
Office of Educational Resources and Research
G 1211 Towsley Center
Ann Arbor, MI 48109
USA

CLINICAL EVALUATION FORM

STUDENT NAME			REPORT COVERS	
			FROM	TO
LAST	FIRST	MIDDLE		
OFFICE USE ONLY:			MO. DAY YR.	MO. DAY YR.

CLERKSHIP

☐ REQUIRED CLERKSHIP

☐ ELECTIVE CLERKSHIP

DEPARTMENT   SECTION   HOSPITAL

EVALUATOR'S NAME

LAST   FIRST INIT.   MIDDLE INIT.

☐ ATTENDING STAFF   ☐ HOUSE STAFF

HISTORY

1 ☐0 NOT OBSERVED	☐1 HISTORY IS INCOMPLETE OR INACCURATE; IMPORTANT INFORMATION IS FREQUENTLY MISSING	☐2 HISTORY IS USUALLY COMPLETE AND ACCURATE BUT OCCASIONALLY IMPORTANT INFORMATION IS MISSING	☐3 HISTORY IS COMPLETE AND ACCURATE; IMPORTANT INFORMATION IS INCLUDED	☐4 HISTORY IS COMPREHENSIVE; INFORMATION IS THOROUGH AND PRECISE; DETAILED FOLLOW UP OBTAINED FOR SIGNIFICANT PROBLEM AREAS

PHYSICAL EXAMINATION (THOROUGHNESS)

2 ☐0 NOT OBSERVED	☐1 DOES NOT CONDUCT COMPLETE EXAM; FAILS TO FOLLOW UP OBVIOUS LEADS; EMPHASIZES MINOR FINDINGS	☐2 GENERALLY CONDUCTS COMPLETE EXAM BUT OCCASIONALLY FAILS TO FOLLOW UP AN OBVIOUS LEAD	☐3 CONDUCTS THOROUGH EXAMINATION; ALL IMPORTANT AREAS ARE FOLLOWED UP	☐4 CONDUCTS THOROUGH EXAMINATION; GATHERS DETAILED INFORMATION REGARDING SPECIFIC AREAS NECESSARY TO OBTAIN DIFFERENTIAL DIAGNOSIS

PHYSICAL EXAMINATION (SKILL & ACCURACY)

3 ☐0 NOT OBSERVED	☐1 MAJOR DEFICIENCIES IN TECHNICAL QUALITY (E.G., CLUMSY OR USES INSTRUMENTS INCORRECTLY)	☐2 MINOR DEFICIENCIES IN TECHNICAL SKILL (E.G., NEEDS TO IMPROVE SPEED OR ACCURACY)	☐3 TECHNICALLY SOUND; USES INSTRUMENTS CORRECTLY; OBTAINS ACCURATE DATA	☐4 PERFORMS TECHNICALLY SOUND, EFFICIENT EXAMINATION EVEN WITH DIFFICULT PROBLEMS; USES INSTRUMENTS CORRECTLY; OBTAINS ACCURATE DATA

APPROPRIATE DIFFERENTIAL DIAGNOSIS/PROBLEM LIST

4 ☐0 NOT OBSERVED	☐1 FREQUENTLY HAS DIFFICULTY USING DATA TO OBTAIN PROBLEM LIST	☐2 OCCASIONALLY HAS DIFFICULTY USING AVAILABLE DATA TO OBTAIN PROBLEM LIST	☐3 EVALUATES AVAILABLE DATA TO OBTAIN PROBLEM LIST	☐4 EFFICIENTLY ANALYZES AVAILABLE DATA; SYNTHESIZES INFORMATION TO ARRIVE AT A CONCISE SUBSTANTIVE PROBLEM LIST

DIAGNOSTIC TEST PLAN

5 ☐0 NOT OBSERVED	☐1 PLAN FOR DIAGNOSTIC TESTS OR CONSULTATION IS INCOMPLETE OR INEFFICIENT; IMPORTANT TESTS ARE FREQUENTLY OVERLOOKED; HAS DIFFICULTY INTERPRETING TEST RESULTS	☐2 PLAN FOR DIAGNOSTIC TESTS OR CONSULTATION IS SOMEWHAT INCOMPLETE OR INEFFICIENT; OCCASIONALLY IMPORTANT TESTS ARE OVERLOOKED; SOMETIMES HAS DIFFICULTY INTERPRETING TEST RESULTS	☐3 PLAN FOR DIAGNOSTIC TESTS OR CONSULTATION IS COMPLETE AND EFFICIENT; IMPORTANT TESTS ARE INCLUDED; INTERPRETS RESULTS CORRECTLY	☐4 PLAN FOR DIAGNOSTIC TESTS OR CONSULTATION IS COMPLETE AND MAXIMIZES INFORMATION GAIN; EFFICIENTLY PLANS ALTERNATIVE DIAGNOSTIC STRATEGY AS RESULTS ARE RECEIVED; INTERPRETS RESULTS CORRECTLY

THERAPEUTIC PROGRAM PLANNING

6 ☐0 NOT OBSERVED	☐1 THERAPEUTIC PROGRAM IS INCOMPLETE OR INACCURATE; IMPORTANT PROCEDURES/ TREATMENTS ARE FREQUENTLY OVERLOOKED	☐2 THERAPEUTIC PROGRAM IS USUALLY COMPLETE AND ACCURATE BUT OCCASIONALLY IMPORTANT PROCEDURES/TREATMENTS ARE OVERLOOKED	☐3 THERAPEUTIC PROGRAM IS COMPLETE AND ACCURATE; IMPORTANT PROCEDURES/ TREATMENTS ARE INCLUDED	☐4 THERAPEUTIC PROGRAM IS COMPREHENSIVE; PLANS ARE THOROUGH AND PRECISE; CAN SUGGEST A VARIETY OF APPROPRIATE ALTERNATIVE PLANS AS RESULTS ARE OBTAINED

PROCEDURAL SKILLS

7 ☐0 NOT OBSERVED	☐1 HAS DIFFICULTY USING PROPER TECHNIQUE (E.G. AWKWARD W/ EQUIPMENT OR BYPASSES ACCEPTED STEPS); FAILS TO ORGANIZE EQUIPMENT PRIOR TO PROCEDURE; HAS DIFFICULTY W/ TIMING/COORDINATION	☐2 OCCASIONALLY HAS DIFFICULTY USING PROPER TECHNIQUE; SOMETIMES FAILS TO ORGANIZE EQUIPMENT PRIOR TO PROCEDURE; MINOR PROBLEMS WITH TIMING OR COORDINATION	☐3 USES PROPER TECHNIQUE; ORGANIZES EQUIPMENT PRIOR TO PROCEDURE; TIMING IS SMOOTH; IS COORDINATED	☐4 USES PROPER TECHNIQUE; ORGANIZES EQUIPMENT PRIOR TO PROCEDURE; TIMING IS PRECISE; PROCEDURES PERFORMED SKILLFULLY AND ADROITLY

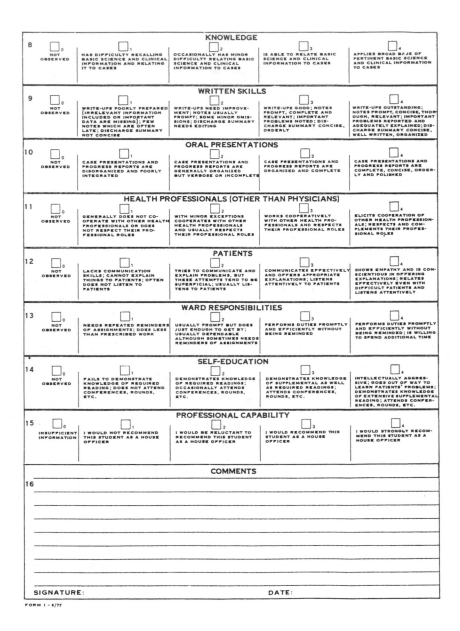

KNOWLEDGE

8

- ☐ 0 — NOT OBSERVED
- ☐ 1 — HAS DIFFICULTY RECALLING BASIC SCIENCE AND CLINICAL INFORMATION AND RELATING IT TO CASES
- ☐ 2 — OCCASIONALLY HAS MINOR DIFFICULTY RELATING BASIC SCIENCE AND CLINICAL INFORMATION TO CASES
- ☐ 3 — IS ABLE TO RELATE BASIC SCIENCE AND CLINICAL INFORMATION TO CASES
- ☐ 4 — APPLIES BROAD BASE OF PERTINENT BASIC SCIENCE AND CLINICAL INFORMATION TO CASES

WRITTEN SKILLS

9

- ☐ 0 — NOT OBSERVED
- ☐ 1 — WRITE-UPS POORLY PREPARED (IRRELEVANT INFORMATION INCLUDED OR IMPORTANT DATA ARE MISSING); FEW NOTES WHICH ARE OFTEN LATE; DISCHARGE SUMMARY NOT CONCISE
- ☐ 2 — WRITE-UPS NEED IMPROVEMENT; NOTES USUALLY PROMPT; SOME MINOR OMISSIONS; DISCHARGE SUMMARY NEEDS EDITING
- ☐ 3 — WRITE-UPS GOOD; NOTES PROMPT, COMPLETE AND RELEVANT; IMPORTANT PROBLEMS NOTED; DISCHARGE SUMMARY CONCISE, ORDERLY
- ☐ 4 — WRITE-UPS OUTSTANDING; NOTES PROMPT, CONCISE, THOROUGH, RELEVANT; IMPORTANT PROBLEMS REPORTED AND ADEQUATELY EXPLAINED; DISCHARGE SUMMARY CONCISE, WELL WRITTEN, ORGANIZED

ORAL PRESENTATIONS

10

- ☐ 0 — NOT OBSERVED
- ☐ 1 — CASE PRESENTATIONS AND PROGRESS REPORTS ARE DISORGANIZED AND POORLY INTEGRATED
- ☐ 2 — CASE PRESENTATIONS AND PROGRESS REPORTS ARE GENERALLY ORGANIZED BUT VERBOSE OR INCOMPLETE
- ☐ 3 — CASE PRESENTATIONS AND PROGRESS REPORTS ARE ORGANIZED AND COMPLETE
- ☐ 4 — CASE PRESENTATIONS AND PROGRESS REPORTS ARE COMPLETE, CONCISE, ORDERLY AND POLISHED

HEALTH PROFESSIONALS (OTHER THAN PHYSICIANS)

11

- ☐ 0 — NOT OBSERVED
- ☐ 1 — GENERALLY DOES NOT COOPERATE WITH OTHER HEALTH PROFESSIONALS OR DOES NOT RESPECT THEIR PROFESSIONAL ROLES
- ☐ 2 — WITH MINOR EXCEPTIONS COOPERATES WITH OTHER HEALTH PROFESSIONALS AND USUALLY RESPECTS THEIR PROFESSIONAL ROLES
- ☐ 3 — WORKS COOPERATIVELY WITH OTHER HEALTH PROFESSIONALS AND RESPECTS THEIR PROFESSIONAL ROLES
- ☐ 4 — ELICITS COOPERATION OF OTHER HEALTH PROFESSIONALS; RESPECTS AND COMPLEMENTS THEIR PROFESSIONAL ROLES

PATIENTS

12

- ☐ 0 — NOT OBSERVED
- ☐ 1 — LACKS COMMUNICATION SKILLS; CANNOT EXPLAIN THINGS TO PATIENTS; OFTEN DOES NOT LISTEN TO PATIENTS
- ☐ 2 — TRIES TO COMMUNICATE AND EXPLAIN PROBLEMS, BUT THESE ATTEMPTS TEND TO BE SUPERFICIAL; USUALLY LISTENS TO PATIENTS
- ☐ 3 — COMMUNICATES EFFECTIVELY AND OFFERS APPROPRIATE EXPLANATIONS; LISTENS ATTENTIVELY TO PATIENTS
- ☐ 4 — SHOWS EMPATHY AND IS CONSCIENTIOUS IN OFFERING EXPLANATIONS; RELATES EFFECTIVELY EVEN WITH DIFFICULT PATIENTS AND LISTENS ATTENTIVELY

WARD RESPONSIBILITIES

13

- ☐ 0 — NOT OBSERVED
- ☐ 1 — NEEDS REPEATED REMINDERS OF ASSIGNMENTS; DOES LESS THAN PRESCRIBED WORK
- ☐ 2 — USUALLY PROMPT BUT DOES JUST ENOUGH TO GET BY; USUALLY DEPENDABLE ALTHOUGH SOMETIMES NEEDS REMINDERS OF ASSIGNMENTS
- ☐ 3 — PERFORMS DUTIES PROMPTLY AND EFFICIENTLY WITHOUT BEING REMINDED
- ☐ 4 — PERFORMS DUTIES PROMPTLY AND EFFICIENTLY WITHOUT BEING REMINDED; IS WILLING TO SPEND ADDITIONAL TIME

SELF-EDUCATION

14

- ☐ 0 — NOT OBSERVED
- ☐ 1 — FAILS TO DEMONSTRATE KNOWLEDGE OF REQUIRED READING; DOES NOT ATTEND CONFERENCES, ROUNDS, ETC.
- ☐ 2 — DEMONSTRATES KNOWLEDGE OF REQUIRED READINGS; OCCASIONALLY ATTENDS CONFERENCES, ROUNDS, ETC.
- ☐ 3 — DEMONSTRATES KNOWLEDGE OF SUPPLEMENTAL AS WELL AS REQUIRED READINGS; ATTENDS CONFERENCES, ROUNDS, ETC.
- ☐ 4 — INTELLECTUALLY AGGRESSIVE; GOES OUT OF WAY TO LEARN PATIENTS' PROBLEMS; DEMONSTRATES KNOWLEDGE OF EXTENSIVE SUPPLEMENTAL READING; ATTENDS CONFERENCES, ROUNDS, ETC.

PROFESSIONAL CAPABILITY

15

- ☐ 0 — INSUFFICIENT INFORMATION
- ☐ 1 — I WOULD NOT RECOMMEND THIS STUDENT AS A HOUSE OFFICER
- ☐ 2 — I WOULD BE RELUCTANT TO RECOMMEND THIS STUDENT AS A HOUSE OFFICER
- ☐ 3 — I WOULD RECOMMEND THIS STUDENT AS A HOUSE OFFICER
- ☐ 4 — I WOULD STRONGLY RECOMMEND THIS STUDENT AS A HOUSE OFFICER

COMMENTS

16

SIGNATURE: DATE:

FORM 1 - 8/77

COMPREHENSIVE ASSESSMENTS (MULTIPLE TASKS)

Type of instrument	Performance	Category of health personnel	Reference Number	Page
Check-list	Diagnostic clinical examination	Physician	9	80
Patient management problem	Diagnosis and management	Physician	10	96
Check-list	History-taking and physical examination	Physician's assistant	11	103
Rating scale	Interviewing	Physician's assistant	12	107
Rating scale	Physical examination	Physician	13	110
Check-list	Physical examination	Physician's assistant	14	114

ASSESSMENT INSTRUMENT 9

I. Check-list: Diagnostic clinical examination (physician)

II. Competences to be assessed:
Gathering, interpreting, and recording data
Communication

III. Specific abilities to be assessed:
1. Ability to obtain relevant medical, social, and psychological histories and record them accurately.
2. Ability to carry out and interpret physical and neurological tests and procedures and record them correctly.
3. Ability to communicate clearly.

IV. Purpose of assessment: summative.
Following a course designed to provide experience in clinical performance, or periodically during an internship.

V. Comments:
Instrument has been pilot-tested with various groups, revised, and various studies of rater reliability have been completed.

VI. Source to contact for further information:
Eta Berner
Associate Professor
Health Professions Education Center for Educational Development
University of Illinois at the Medical Center
808 South Wood Street
Chicago, IL 60612
USA

PERFORMANCE OF DIAGNOSTIC CLINICAL EXAMINATION

INSTRUCTIONS TO OBSERVERS:

This checklist should be filled out as follows: Place a check in the appropriate white (NOT SHADED) space that describes the student's behavior.

INQUIRED ABOUT ITEM — if student asks only one question pertaining to item

FAILED TO EXPAND UPON ITEM WHEN NECESSARY — if student does not probe further after initial question when it is judged that he should do so

DONE CORRECTLY — if student performs all parts of the item in the proper manner

DONE INCORRECTLY — if student performs all parts of the item, but does not use proper technique or does not do it in enough detail

NOT DONE, OMITTED ITEM — if student does not perform the item

RECORDED ACCURATELY & COMPLETELY — if student's written record is an accurate interpretation of the data

RECORDED INACCURATELY &/or INCOMPLETELY — if student records erroneous information or not enough information

NOT RECORDED — if the item was performed, but does not appear in the student's write-up

N.A. under PERFORMANCE — if the observer feels the item is NOT APPLICABLE or NOT APPROPRIATE for the given student or patient

N.A. under RECORD OF EXAMINATION — if for any reason student did not perform the item

The spaces labelled COMMENTS are to be used for any additional comments, clarifications, or explanations that the observer wishes to make.

HISTORY

PRESENT ILLNESS	PERFORMANCE						WRITTEN RECORD			
	COL. #	INQUIRED ABOUT ITEM (1)	FAILED TO EXPAND UPON ITEM WHEN NECESSARY (2)	OMITTED ITEM (3)	N.A. (4)	COL. #	RECORDED ACCURATELY & COMPLETELY (1)	RECORDED INACCURATELY &/or INCOMPLETELY (2)	NOT RECORDED (3)	N.A. (4)
1. Chief complaint in patient's own words	(11)					(24)				
2. Duration of each complaint	(12)					(25)				
3. Location of the symptom	(13)					(26)				
4. Site of origin of the symptom	(14)					(27)				
5. Severity of the symptom	(15)					(28)				
6. Character of the symptom	(16)					(29)				
7. Factors relieving the symptom	(17)					(30)				
8. Factors that make the symptom worse	(18)					(31)				
9. How the symptom started (abruptly, gradually, intermittently)	(19)					(32)				
10. Radiation of the symptom	(20)					(33)				
11. Onset and course of the symptom complex	(21)					(34)				
12. Questions pertinent to other complaints that are discovered	(22)									
13. Ask the patient about present illness in a flexible way without a checklist of questions	(23)									

2

OTHER DATA	COL. #	INQUIRED ABOUT ITEM (1)	FAILED TO EXPAND UPON ITEM WHEN NECESSARY (2)	OMITTED ITEM (3)	N.A. (4)	COL. #	RECORDED ACCURATELY & COMPLETELY (1)	RECORDED INACCURATELY &/or INCOMPLETELY (2)	NOT RECORDED (3)	N.A. (4)
14. Past medical history	(35)					(49)				
15. Home and family situation and its impact on illness	(36)					(50)				
16. Environment (including occupational environment) and its impact on illness	(37)					(51)				
17. Patient's age	(38)					(52)				
18. Geographic origins	(39)					(53)				
19. Occupational history	(40)					(54)				
20. Smoking (current and in the past)	(41)					(55)				
21. Alcohol intake (current and in the past)	(42)					(56)				
22. Drug usage	(43)					(57)				
23. Allergies (generally)	(44)					(58)				
24. Allergy to penicillin	(45)					(59)				
25. Family history	(46)					(60)				
26. Venereal disease	(47)					(61)				
27. Other infectious diseases	(48)					(62)				

COMMENTS:

3

REVIEW OF SYSTEMS	COL. #	INQUIRED ABOUT ITEM (1)	FAILED TO EXPAND UPON ITEM WHEN NECESSARY (2)	OMITTED ITEM (3)	N.A. (4)	COL. #	RECORD ACCURATELY & COMPLETELY (1)	RECORDED INACCURATELY &/or INCOMPLETELY (2)	NOT RECORDED (3)	N.A. (4)
28. Endocrine	(63)					(71)				
29. Respiratory	(64)					(72)				
30. Cardiovascular	(65)					(73)				
31. Gastrointestinal	(66)					(74)				
32. Genitourinary	(67)					(75)				
33. Neurological	(68)					(76)				
34. Musculoskeletal	(69)					(77)				
35. Questions pertinent to other complaints that are discovered in the review of systems	(70)					(78)				

COMMENTS:

Dup. 1-5
Col. 6-7 = 02
Dup. 8-9

PSYCHOLOGICAL HISTORY

	COL.# INQUIRED ABOUT ITEM (1)	FAILED TO EXPAND UPON ITEM WHEN NECESSARY (2)	OMITTED ITEM (3)	N.A. (4)	COL.#	RECORDED ACCURATELY & COMPLETELY (1)	RECORDED INACCURATELY &/or INCOMPLETELY (2)	NOT RECORDED (3)	N.A. (4)
36. Patient's verbal behavior (garrulous, reticent, quiet)					(11)				
37. Patient's non-verbal behavior					(12)				
38. Patient's mood					(13)				
39. Appropriateness of patient's mood					(14)				
40. Patient's major coping mechanisms to adapt to illness					(15)				
41. Effectiveness of coping mechanisms (patient's state of psychological equilibrium)					(16)				
42. Reliability of the patient					(17)				
43. Patient's orientation					(18)				
44. Presence or absence of underlying psychiatric syndrome					(19)				

INTERVIEW SKILLS

During the interview how often did the student:

	Col.#	MOST OF THE TIME (1)	ABOUT HALF THE TIME (2)	SELDOM (3)	N.A. (4)
45. Allow patient to talk without interrupting him unnecessarily?	(20)				
46. Allow patient to tell his story in his own words?	(21)				
47. Ask open-ended questions when appropriate?	(22)				
48. Use language appropriate to patient's ability to understand?	(23)				
49. Maintain control of the direction of the interview?	(24)				
50. Refrain from intimidating patient in an attempt to get information?	(25)				
51. Intervene with appropriate responses when patient was unable to supply relevant information?	(26)				
52. Obtain information in an efficient manner?	(27)				

5

PHYSICAL EXAM

	PERFORMANCE					WRITTEN RECORD			
GENERAL INSPECTION	COL. #	DONE CORRECTLY (1)	DONE INCORRECTLY (2)	NOT DONE (3)	N.A. (4)	COL. #	RECORDED ACCURATELY & COMPLETELY (1)	RECORDED INACCURATELY &/or INCOMPLETELY (2)	NOT RECORDED (3)	N.A. (4)
1. General state of health (acute or chronic illness, nourishment)						(30)				
2. Estimation of somatic age (older, younger, same as stated age)						(31)				
3. Description of physical attitudes of patient (sitting, lying, etc.)						(32)				
4. Description of body habitus						(33)				
5. Description of condition of patient's skin						(34)				
VITAL SIGNS										
6. Take blood pressure in both arms	(28)					(35)				
7. Palpate pulse	(29)					(36)				
8. Measure respiration rate						(37)				

6

HEAD	COL #	DONE CORRECTLY (1)	DONE INCORRECTLY (2)	NOT DONE (3)	N.A. (4)	COL #	RECORDED ACCURATELY & COMPLETELY (1)	RECORDED INACCURATELY &/or INCOMPLETELY (2)	NOT RECORDED (3)	N.A. (4)
9. Inspect head	(38)					(52)				
10. Inspect scalp	(39)					(53)				
11. Palpate scalp	(40)					(54)				
12. Inspect the face	(41)					(55)				
13. Inspect the ear canal and tympanic membrane bilaterally	(42)					(56)				
14. Estimate visual acuity (reading print, eye chart, other standard)	(43)					(57)				
15. Inspect external ocular structures (lids, conjunctive, cornea)	(44)					(58)				
16. Observe pupillary response to light and accomodation	(45)					(59)				
17. Evaluate ocular muscle function and eye alignment	(46)					(60)				
18. Inspect the lens and retina with ophthalmoscope	(47)					(61)				
19. Inspect the nose	(48)					(62)				
20. Inspect the entire mouth for lesions (including lips, buccal mucosa, tongue, subglossal area, tonsils, posterior pharynx, dentition, gingivee, palate)	(49)					(63)				
21. Palpate all observable lesions in the mouth	(50)									
22. Have the patient remove dental appliance (if present) before examination	(51)									

7

Dup. 1-5
Col. 6-7 = 03
Dup. 8-9

NECK	COL. #	DONE CORRECTLY (1)	DONE INCORRECTLY (2)	NOT DONE (3)	N.A. (4)	COL. #	RECORDED ACCURATELY & COMPLETELY (1)	RECORDED INACCURATELY &/or INCOMPLETELY (2)	NOT RECORDED (3)	N.A. (4)
23. Palpate for lymph nodes	(11)					(20)				
24. Palpate for parotid gland	(12)					(21)				
25. Palpate for submandibular gland	(13)					(22)				
26. Palpate thyroid without swallowing	(14)					(23)				
27. Palpate thyroid with swallowing	(15)					(24)				
28. Inspect and palpate supraclavicular area	(16)					(25)				
29. Determine range of motion of cervical spine	(17)					(26)				
30. Inspect neck veins	(18)					(27)				
31. Auscultate carotids	(19)					(28)				

COMMENTS:

CHEST & BREASTS	COL. #	DONE CORRECTLY (1)	DONE INCORRECTLY (2)	NOT DONE (3)	N.A. (4)	COL. #	RECORDED ACCURATELY & COMPLETELY (1)	RECORDED INACCURATELY &/or INCOMPLETELY (2)	NOT RECORDED (3)	N.A. (4)
32. Inspect thorax anteriorly & posteriorly during inspiration & expiration	(29)					(45)				
33. Palpate ribs and thorax	(30)					(46)				
34. Percuss the chest	(31)					(47)				
35. Auscultate all areas of thorax (supraclavicular, subclavicular, anterior, posterior, lateral)	(32)					(48)				
36. Test for tactile and/or vocal fremitus	(33)					(49)				
37. Examine breasts in both sitting and lying position	(34)					(50)				
38. Inspect breasts visually in all positions (normal, with active elevation of arms, leaning forward)	(35)					(51)				
39. Palpate entire breast bilaterally (nipple, areolar and subareolar area, breast proper, tail of Spence, axilla)	(36)					(52)				
40. Attempt to express material from nipple	(37)					(53)				
41. Examine axilla with passive motion of the arm (abduction)	(38)					(54)				
42. Redrape breasts at completion of exam	(39)					(55)				
43. Palpate cardiac area for heaves, thrills	(40)					(56)				
44. Determination of cardiac size by percussion	(41)					(57)				
45. Auscultate all areas of transmitted cardiac sounds (pulmonary, aortic, mitral, tricuspid)	(42)									
46. Trace transmission pattern of a murmur if present	(43)									
47. Observe murmur in all positions (sitting, leaning forward, lying down)	(44)									

9

ABDOMINAL EXAM	COL. #	DONE CORRECTLY (1)	DONE INCORRECTLY (2)	NOT DONE (3)	N.A. (4)	COL. #	RECORDED ACCURATELY & COMPLETELY (1)	RECORDED INACCURATELY &/or INCOMPLETELY (2)	NOT RECORDED (3)	N.A. (4)
48. Inspect abdomen including both flanks and groin	(58)					(66)				
49. Presence of surgical scars or lesions						(67)				
50. Auscultate before manipulation or palpation	(59)									
51. Description of bowel sounds						(68)				
52. Percuss the abdomen	(60)									
53. Palpate the abdomen systematically	(61)									
54. Description of tonus of abdominal musculature						(69)				
55. Presence or absence of abdominal masses						(70)				
56. Position patient for palpation of liver and spleen	(62)									
57. Percuss the liver	(63)									
58. Description of liver size						(71)				
59. Description of liver consistency						(72)				
60. Palpability of spleen						(73)				
61. Examine for CVA tenderness	(64)					(74)				
62. Palpate the abdomen thoroughly without being rough	(65)									

10

Dup. 1-5
Col. 6-7 = 04
Dup. 8-9

GROIN	COL #	DONE CORRECTLY (1)	DONE INCORRECTLY (2)	NOT DONE (3)	N.A. (4)	COL #	RECORDED ACCURATELY & COMPLETELY (1)	RECORDED INACCURATELY &/or INCOMPLETELY (2)	NOT RECORDED (3)	N.A. (4)
63. Examine for hernia	(11)					(14)				
64. Palpate over fossa ovalis bilaterally (palpate for femoral hernia)	(12)					(15)				
65. Palpate external inguinal ring bilaterally	(13)					(16)				

COMMENTS:

11

EXTREMITIES	COL. #	DONE CORRECTLY (1)	DONE INCORRECTLY (2)	NOT DONE (3)	N.A. (4)	COL. #	RECORDED ACCURATELY & COMPLETELY (1)	RECORDED INACCURATELY &/or INCOMPLETELY (2)	NOT RECORDED (3)	N.A. (4)
66. Determine range of motion of elbow	(17)					(28)				
67. Determine range of motion of forearm	(18)					(29)				
68. Determine range of motion of wrist and fingers	(19)					(30)				
69. Test for strength of abduction of shoulder	(20)					(31)				
70. Test for strength of flexion of elbow	(21)					(32)				
71. Test for strength of grip bilaterally	(22)					(33)				
72. Inspect the fingernails	(23)					(34)				
73. Inspect the entire lower extremities (all parts of legs, thighs, feet, ankles, toes, between toes)	(24)					(35)				
74. Description of muscle mass in lower extremities						(36)				
75. Description of condition of the skin						(37)				
76. Presence or absence of hair						(38)				
77. Presence or absence of deformities						(39)				
78. Description of the toe nails						(40)				
79. Palpate for differences in skin temperature	(25)									
80. Examine all pulses bilaterally (femoral, popliteal, posterior, tibial, dorsalis pedis)	(26)									
81. Description of strength of pulses						(41)				
82. Determine range of motion of hips, knees and ankles	(27)					(42)				

12

BACK	COL. #	DONE CORRECTLY (1)	DONE INCORRECTLY (2)	NOT DONE (3)	N.A. (4)	COL. #	RECORDED ACCURATELY & COMPLETELY (1)	RECORDED INACCURATELY &/or INCOMPLETELY (2)	NOT RECORDED (3)	N.A. (4)
83. Properly drape patient	(43)									
84. Instruct patient to stand on hard floor	(44)									
85. Inspect patient's spine	(45)					(49)				
86. Instruct patient to walk barefooted and record gait	(46)					(50)				
87. Instruct patient to walk on tiptoes and record presence or absence of weakness	(47)					(51)				
88. Instruct patient to walk on heels and record presence or absence of weakness	(48)					(52)				

COMMENTS:

13

NEUROLOGICAL EXAM	COL. #	DONE CORRECTLY (1)	DONE INCORRECTLY (2)	NOT DONE (3)	N.A. (4)	COL. #	RECORDED ACCURATELY & COMPLETELY (1)	RECORDED INACCURATELY &/or INCOMPLETELY (2)	NOT RECORDED (3)	N.A. (4)
89. Patient's speech						(66)				
90. Masseter compression; jaw opening; facial sensation (V)	(53)					(67)				
91. Facial muscles (VII)	(54)					(68)				
92. Hearing (VIII) (Weber and Rinne)	(55)					(69)				
93. Swallowing; gag response; palatal movement (IX and X)	(56)					(70)				
94. Shrug shoulders (XI)	(57)					(71)				
95. Tongue movement (XII)	(58)					(72)				
96. Test for all deep tendon reflexes (patellar, triceps, achilles, biceps)	(59)					(73)				
97. Test for abdominal reflex	(60)					(74)				
98. Test for pathological reflexes (example: Babinski; clonus)	(61)					(75)				
99. Test vibratory sense	(62)					(76)				
100. Test for neurosensory loss	(63)					(77)				
101. Test cerebellar function (finger-nose; heel-shin; rapid alternating movements)	(64)					(78)				
102. Test proprioception (examples: Rhomberg, position sense in great toe)	(65)					(79)				

14

Dup. 1-5
Col. 6-7 = 05
Dup. 8-9

RELATIONSHIP TO PATIENT

	COL. #	YES (1)	NO (2)	N.A. (3)
103. Did the student inquire as to the patient's feelings about his present illness?	(11)			
104. Did the student inquire as to how well the patient understands his present illness?	(12)			

How often during the history and physical exam did the student:

	COL. #	MOST OF THE TIME (1)	ABOUT HALF THE TIME (2)	SELDOM (3)	N.A. (4)
105. Deal with patient's expressed questions and concerns?	(13)				
106. Deal with patient's non-verbally communicated concerns (trembling, signs of pain, etc.)?	(14)				
107 Refrain from doing or saying anything to unnecessarily arouse patient's anxiety?	(15)				
108. Display appropriate affect?	(16)				
109. Present self in professional manner (verbal and non-verbal behavior)?	(17)				

What specific problems did this patient pose for the student in terms of interview and examination skills he/she could or could not have demonstrated? (Circle appropriate number.)

110. Patient was highly cooperative, volunteered information freely; was able to deal with own feelings freely and spontaneously.   1 2 3 4 5 (18)   Patient was highly uncooperative and/or unable to respond; information extremely difficult to elicit, unable or unwilling to deal with feelings.

111. Patient was cooperative during physical exam.   1 2 3 4 5 (19)   Patient was uncooperative during physical exam.

15

ASSESSMENT INSTRUMENT 10

I. Patient management problem: Diagnosis and management (physician

II. Competences to be assessed:
Data interpretation
Diagnosis
Treatment-planning
Patient education

III. Specific abilities to be assessed:
1. Ability to diagnose a health problem correctly, given case history and examination data.
2. Ability to identify the essential problems in a case.
3. Ability to develop appropriate plans for treatment and patient education.

IV. Purpose of assessment: summative.
Test has been used as a comprehensive examination at the end of a sequence of courses in the third year of medical school.

V. Comments:
Instrument has been evaluated by both faculty and students by means of written feedback reactions. No statistical data are available, however.

VI. Source to contact for further information:
Dr James P. Hale
Coordinator of Instructional Design and Evaluation
Office of Educational Resources
University of South Dakota Medical School
Vermillion, SD 57069
USA

PATIENT MANAGEMENT PROBLEM

Note for students

In the morning, the student will read a short case history and physical examination data from which he/she is to develop (*a*) an initial problem list that includes a differential diagnosis for each problem, (*b*) an assessment of the situation, (*c*) an appropriate diagnostic plan, treatment plan, and patient education plan. This should take approximately 30 minutes. The examiner and student will meet together and the examiner will allow the student to proceed with his/her diagnostic plan. He/she will give the student results from requested laboratory tests. In addition, the examiner will question the student's approach and guide the student into the right general area by asking pertinent questions. At the completion of this session, the examiner will give all remaining data to the student which he/she has not asked for but which is considered appropriate or necessary for the diagnosis and treatment of the patient. The session will take one hour.

On the next morning, the areas mentioned above are covered with the student, as well as the references utilized by the student in working on the problem. More credit should be given for references from current journals than for those from textbooks. The student should (*a*) present written progress notes on each identified problem in SOAP[1] format, (*b*) be prepared to give an oral explanation of the disease processes involved and justification for diagnosis and treatment, (*c*) prepare a bibliography of not less than 5 or more than 15 of the most pertinent references, including consultants. The student may bring reference material to the examination including articles, textbooks, reports from consultants, or other written materials he or others have prepared. The examiner will be the same for both days for a given student working on a specific problem. The instructor will read the student's progress notes and bibliography and orally examine the student regarding his progress notes, bibliography, understanding, logic, and problem-solving abilities.

The student will discuss the case with a physician-examiner for approximately one hour, and will be able to seek additional data from him/her as well. The student will have the afternoon and evening to pursue the patient management problems using any and all available resources i.e., books, journals, consultants, fellow students, etc. On the next morning, he/she will spend one hour with the examiner discussing the case.

The forms that will be used to evaluate performance on the patient management problem are attached. Exceptional = 5, good = 3, adequate = 2, marginal = 1, unacceptable = 0, not evaluated = omit. The minimum passing level for the patient management problem is:

(1) a *maximum* of two marginal ratings and *at least* an adequate rating for both days;[2] and

(2) a *minimum* mean value of 1.75 for
(*a*) all 9 ratings for the first day,
(*b*) all 10 ratings for the second day.

---

[1] S = subjective; O = objective; A = assessment; P = plans.
[2] Any one rating of "unacceptable" indicates failure.

RATING FORM FOR THE ORAL PROBLEM-SOLVING PORTION OF THE COMPREHENSIVE EVALUATION

First day

Student _____ Date_____

Examiner(s) _____ Problem No._____

Items for evaluation	Exceptional	Good	Adequate	Marginal	Unacceptable	Not evaluated
Adequacy of initial problem list						
Adequacy of diagnostic plan						
Adequacy of treatment plan						
Adequacy of patient education plan						
Ability to obtain appropriate diagnostic data						
Ability to explain his/her problem-solving strategy						
Fund of related basic science knowledge						
Fund of related clinical science knowledge						
Overall performance						

Comments (required):

Second day

Student _____ Date _____

Examiner(s) _____ Problem No. _____

Items for evaluation	Exceptional	Good	Adequate	Marginal	Unacceptable	Not evaluated
Adequacy of resources utilized						
Adequacy of current problem list and progress notes						
Adequacy of current diagnosis						
Adequacy of current treatment plan						
Adequacy of current patient education plan						
Ability to explain his/her problem-solving strategy						
Fund of related basic science knowledge						
Fund of related clinical science knowledge						
Overall progress from previous day						
Overall performance today						

Comments (required):

PROBLEM NO. 7

Name: M.K.—123 *Address*: Wagner, SD *Age*: 15 years *Sex*: Female *Civil state*: Single *Occupation*: Student
Race: White Admitted: 12/75 (Yankton)

This young teenager presented with:

Chief complaint: Headaches, nausea, vomiting—2 months' duration.
Informants: Mother plus patient—both appeared reliable.
Present illness: The patient was apparently well until 2 months prior to admission when the patient developed headaches, usually in the right or left frontal area, pounding in character, lasting 3–4 hours, occurring 3–4 times per week and associated with nausea and vomiting. The headaches may occur at any time of the day. There is no numbness or weakness on either side associated with the headaches.
The patient has had some nose bleeds the preceeding summer.
Medication: None
Family, developmental-social history: Patient has a sister who has one hip socket missing and also has had some form of kidney problem—type unknown. Otherwise negative.
Past history: The mother relates that her daughter has a history of frequent urinary tract infections, but her daughter is not a complainer and would not complain unless the infections were really bad. The patient was hospitalized for 10 days for urinary tract infection at another institution 2 years ago. No X-ray studies were performed and laboratory values were unknown.

Review of systems: Non-contributory except for:
1. Lack of energy for the past 5–6 months
2. Menarche—age 13 years—regular cycle
Physical examination: height 64½ inches (25–50 percentile); weight 114 pounds (25–50 percentile); heart rate 18; pulse 72; temperature 98.6° (oral); blood pressure 188/120 right arm lying, 170/120 left arm lying, 200/130 right leg lying, 190/130 left leg lying.
The patient is a 15-year-old white female who is well developed, well nourished and in no acute distress. She is oriented to time, place and person and is pleasant and cooperative.
Head: Normocephalic without bruits.
EENT: Ear canals are clear; tympanic membranes normal color and intact. Dental hygiene good. Throat showed no inflammation or lesions. Sclerae-conjunctivae clear. Extraocular movements normal without nystagmus. Pupils, round, regular, equal, react to light. Funduscopic—normal.
Chest: Breasts: Early prepubertal
    Lungs: Clear to auscultation and palpation, percussion.
    Cardiac: Rate is regular. Grade I/VI systolic murmur along left sternal border at 2nd left interspace with radiation into left carotid.
Abdomen: Soft, tympanitic with active bowel sounds. No organomegaly or other masses. Femoral pulses are full and equal bilaterally.
Genitourinary: Externally normal female.
Rectal: Not done.
Extremities: Full range of motion without deformities.

Neurological: Cranial nerves I–XII were intact. Muscle strength and tone good in upper and lower extremities. Abduction, adduction, internal and external rotation, extension and flexion good.
Reflexes: Biceps, triceps, brachial radialis, patellas, Achilles are 2–3 + bilaterally. Plantar reflexes were downgoing bilaterally.
Gait and coordination: Intact-to rapid alternating movements in the upper and lower extremities. Finger to nose was done bilaterally without difficulty and the patient was able to draw a triangle without difficulty with her foot. Gait: normal (toe, heel, tandem, ordinary gait). Romberg: negative.

Admission-*complete blood count (CBC)* + *urinalysis*
CBC   Hemoglobin (Hgb) 8.4 g/100 ml
           Hematocrit (Hct) 26%
           White blood cells (WBC)—4900 with 2% bands, 52% segments, 1% basophils, 1% eosinophils, 42% lymphocytes, and 2% monocytes.
Urine   pH 6.0
           Specific gravity 1.014
           Albumin 3 +
           Sugar $\overline{0}$
           Acetone $\overline{0}$
           WBC 1–2/high power field (hpf)
           Red blood cells (RBC) 15–20/hpf
           No crystals or casts

PATIENT MANAGEMENT PROBLEM

(FOR EXAMINER ONLY)

Patient: M.K.—123

Screening lab. data in addition to complete blood count and urinalysis:

Nà 137, K 4.8, Cl 105, *CO_2 content 14, pH 7.35

Profile: *Ca 8.6, *P 6.9, glucose 120, *blood urea nitrogen (BUN) 58, uric acid 7.5, cholesterol 245, total serum protein 6.5, albumin 3.7, total bilirubin 0.5, *Alk. phosphatase 125, LDH 260, SGOT 20.

* Abnormal

Essential problems:

1. Hypertension (with headaches, nausea, vomiting)

2. Chronic renal disease
   - a. Proteinuria
   - b. Hematuria, microscopic
   - c. Azotemia
   - d. Hypocalcemia, mild
   - e. Hyperphosphatemia
   - f. Acidosis (low CO_2 content, borderline low pH)
   - g. Anemia

3. Urinary tract infection—past history

If the student does not have the profile prior to being asked the problem list then the essential problems would be:

1. Hypertension (with headaches, nausea, vomiting)
2. Anemia
3. Proteinuria
4. Hematuria, microscopic
5. Urinary tract infection, past history of

Eventually the student should arrive at a diagnosis which should essentially be:

1. Reflux nephropathy, bilateral
2. Chronic renal disease, with associated:
   - a. hypertension
   - b. secondary hyperparathyroidism
   - c. anemia
   - d. acidosis
   - e. azotemia
   - f. proteinuria and hematuria
   - g. infection

Essential problems

1. Hypertension—The student has received information via lectures that hypertension in a teenager in general falls into 2 groups. Essential for white males, black males, and females. Secondary: white females. Therefore, he should quickly decide that the hypertension is secondary to some underlying disease process and most likely will pick renal artery stenosis as the first option, though in actuality with the anemia, proteinuria, and hematuria available from the initial lab. data, the student should rather say: Chronic renal disease—?etiology—perhaps glomerulo-nephritis or pyelonephritis.

The student may however start off with a differential diagnosis of hypertension which would probably include the following:

1. Coarctation of aorta—Ruled out by lower extremity blood pressure.
2. Pheochromocytoma—No lab. studies were done—since renal disease was found.
3. Hyperthyroidism—No clinical evidence. No lab. studies done.
4. Hyperaldosteronism—No alkalosis or hypokalemia.
5. Brain tumor—No projectile vomiting, no papilledema.
6. Renal artery stenosis—No abdominal bruits. Peripheral blood renin levels 5 hours post-Lasix (furosemide) = 0.4 ng ml h (normal = 0.4—4.5 ng ml h).

7. Chronic renal disease
   a. Glomerulonephritis—red blood cells in urine
   Necessary lab. data: Intravenous pyelography (IVP) (available for student interpretation). Interpretation: Bilateral function with slow uptake; kidneys equal in size, both small; suggesting bilateral renal disease, possibly chronic glomerulonephritis.
   b. Pyelonephritis—Small kidneys on IVP
   Necessary lab. data: Urine culture—negative
   c. Reflux nephropathy
   Necessary lab. data: Voiding cystourethrogram (available for student interpretation)—Bilateral ureterorenal reflux on voiding.
   Consultation: May consult radiologist regarding X-rays. May consult nephrologist regarding reflux nephropathy versus pyelonephritis. May consult *Kidney International*, Supplement 4, August 1975, for a discussion of reflux nephropathy.
   Initial Treatment: May select any of a variety of antihypertensive agents, for which the student should know site of action, onset of action, dose, contraindications, and reactions.
   Thiazides – Renin stimulating by virtue of decreasing plasma volume works in distal tubule loop of Henle. Onset of action—1 hour (oral). Dose: $50 \text{ mg/m}^2/\text{day}$ orally in 2 divided doses. Contraindications: Renin type hypertension. Reactions: Primarily hematopoietic, plus alkalosis, hypokalemia, etc.
   Reserpine – Renin-inhibitor. Action at nerve ending—depletes catecholamine stores. Onset of action—3–4 days (oral), 3–4 hours (IM). Dose: 0.1–0.2 mg twice daily to start. Contraindication: Peptic ulcer, mental depression. Reactions: Nasal obstruction, diarrhea, nightmares, depression.
   Alpha-methyl DOPA – Renin-inhibitor—Inhibits catecholamine synthesis. Onset of action—2 hours (oral, IV). Dose: 10 mg/kg/day in 2–3 divided doses (oral), 20–40 mg/kg/day in 2–4 divided doses (IV). Reactions: Postural hypotension, hepatitis and hemolytic anemia, drug fever.
   Hydralazine – Dilatation of arterioles and decreased peripheral resistance—acts on arterioles. Onset: 3 hours (oral) 10–20 minutes (IV). Dose: 0.75 mg/kg/24 hours in 4 doses (oral), 1.7 3.5 mg/kg/24 hours in 4–6 divided doses (IV). Reactions: tachycardia, palpitation, headache, diarrhea, lupus syndrome.
In the patient under discussion 2 drugs were used: hydrochlorothiazide 25 mg twice daily orally plus reserpine 0.2 mg twice daily orally with BP control at about 130–140/80.

2. Chronic renal disease
   a. Proteinuria
   Necessary lab.: Repeat urinalysis revealed 3–4 × proteinuria. 24-hour urine protein not done.
   b. Hematuria—microscopic—persistent 8–10 red blood cells/high power field
   c. Azotemia
   Necessary lab.: Repeat BUN 35, 58
   Creatinine clearance = 11.3 ml/min (Serum creatinine = 3.3 mg%)
   d. Hypocalcemia, mild
   e. Hyperphosphatemia—Repeat 7.2
   f. Acidosis – Repeat CO_2 content = 16 meq/L, pH 7.38
   g. Anemia
   Necessary lab.: Retic count 1.9% Direct Coomb's negative. Indirect Coomb's negative. Red cell indices: mean cell volume 81 (87–97), mean cell hemoglobin content 35.5% (31–35), mean cell hemoglobin 28 (28 31), repeat hematocrit 24%.
3. Urinary tract infection— past history
   Necessary lab.: Repeat urine culture—100 000 *Escherichia coli.*
The student should reach the diagnosis as noted above.

The treatment of the chronic renal disease with the associated problems should be:

a. Hypertension – as noted above.
b. Secondary hyperparathyroidism
   (a) Amphojel (aluminum hydroxide gel)—To block phosphate absorption. Dose will vary—started at 600 mg three times a day.
   Follow-up reveals P of 5.7 (2 months post-hospital).
c. Anemia—no therapy. The use of $FeSO_4$ is not indicated—no iron deficiency; rather hemolysis plus poor marrow function.
d. Acidosis—Use of $NaHCO_3$ started at 1200 mg three times a day. Follow-up CO_2 27 meq L.
e. Azotemia 20 g protein diet
f. Proteinuria +hematuria—No treatment.

The reflux nephropathy might be handled:
   (a) Surgically with reimplantation
Consultant-urologist. Actually we decided on 6 months conservative medical management
   (b) Medical: (1) Treat infections
                (2) Double to triple voiding
                (3) Follow biochemical lab. values.
g. Urinary tract infection
   (a) Treatment—ampicillin—bacteria sensitive to this drug which is not contraindicated in the face of chronic renal failure.

Patient-family education revolves around the problem of chronic renal disease with hypertension and failure. The areas that must be stressed are:

1. Control of the hypertension—hypertension itself can intensify the renal disease and failure.
2. Dietary management to alleviate or prevent as far as possible the effects of uremia.
3. Amphojel to prevent or control the bone effect of secondary hyperparathyroidism. Later Vitamin D or one of its metabolites may need to be added to the regimen.
4. Bicarbonate use to provide body with buffer so metabolism is normal.
5. The fact that the child has chronic renal failure and that our therapy is directed toward aiding the kidneys to maintain as far as possible body homeostasis, but that this therapy will not reverse the disease process.
6. Control of urinary tract infection because of the easy accessibility to the kidneys as a consequence of the bilateral reflux.
7. The possible use of surgery to stop the reflux, but the possibility that it may not or that ureteral obstruction could occur post-operatively. Further that is unlikely to reverse the process.
8. The strong likelihood of dialysis and renal transplantation in the future—estimated as the time when the creatinine clearance is 5 ml min 1.73 m².

ASSESSMENT INSTRUMENT 11

I. Check-list: History-taking and physical examination (physician's assistant)

II. Competence to be assessed:
   Data-gathering

III. Specific ability to be assessed:
   Ability to elicit comprehensive medical-social history.

IV. Purpose of assessment:
   Used as a mid-term evaluation in a course in medical history-taking for physician's assistants.

V. Comments:
   Totally concerned with data or content, and not with technique. Criteria are simply P (present) or, if any of the listed points are omitted, A (absent). No evaluation data are available.

VI. Source to contact for further information:
   Martha Duhamel
   MEDEX Northwest
   University of Washington
   Seattle, WA
   USA

HISTORY-TAKING EVALUATION

Student's name _____
Evaluator _____
Date _____

Interview critique sheet (content)

Note. *P* = present, *A* = absent for each of the following:

Opening remarks
_____Greeting (name)
_____Introduce self
_____Purpose explained
_____Time estimated
_____Consent obtained
_____Attention to comfort and privacy
Comments:

Opening question (verbatim):

_____*Identification data*

Patient profile
_____Cultural (if not in ID data)
_____Marital status (if not in ID data)
_____Occupation (if not in ID data)
_____Personal support system
_____Financial situation
_____Self-understanding
Comments:

Chief complaint
_____Brief statement of patient's specific reason for seeking medical care
_____Duration of complaint
Comments:

History of present illness
_____Onset—time
_____   —sudden or gradual
_____Duration
_____Description
_____   —location
_____   —radiation
_____   —severity
_____Factors increasing
_____Factors decreasing
_____Review of systems
_____Effect on patient
_____Medications/treatment
_____Family history
Comments:

Past medical history
_____Covers illnesses_____place_____date_____doctor_____sequelae
_____Covers surgeries_____place_____date_____doctor_____sequelae
_____Covers hospitalizations_____place_____date_____doctor_____sequelae
Comments:

Medication
_____Asks about current medication
_____Clarifies dosage schedule
_____Asks about vitamins and over-the-counter medicaments
Comments:

Allergies and drug reactions
_____Asks about allergies
_____Asks about drug reactions
_____Clarifies "type" of reaction if drug allergy is positive
Comments:

Interview critique sheet (contd.)

Health data
_____Physical exam._____date_____result
_____Chest X-ray_____date_____result
_____ECG_____date_____result
_____TB skin test_____date_____result
_____Pap smear_____date_____result
_____Immunizations
_____Transfusions
Comments:

Habits
_____Coffee
_____Tobacco
_____Alcohol

Family history
_____Asks about parents and children and sibs
_____Asks list of key diseases (heart disease, cancer, stroke, etc.)

Review of systems
_____Asks questions about each system
_____Asks questions in such a way that the patient can understand and doesn't use medical jargon
(Check questions asked on attached review of systems sheet)

Closing
_____Open-ended question at end ("Anything else you'd like to mention that would be helpful for me to know?")
_____Summation
_____Next step
_____Thank you

REVIEW OF SYSTEMS
Patient data base

Name of patient_____

Check if there is no significant problem: *circle* if there is a significant problem and *record* details or note "PMH" (previous medical history) if recorded elsewhere. Items not marked are assumed to be not examined.

General	
Weight change	Fever, chills
Weakness	Fatigue
Sweating, nightsweats	
Skin	
Nail changes	Itching
Rash, eruptions	
Head	
Headache	Trauma
Eyes	
Vision, glasses	Blurring
Photophobia	Diplopia
Inflammation	Scotoma
Ears/nose/mouth	
Pain	Discharge
Deafness	Tinnitus
Vertigo	Hearing
Sinusitis	Polyps
Epistaxis	Obstruction
Sores	Postnasal drip
Teeth	Sore throat
Taste	Gums
Breath	Dentures
Respiratory	
Wheezing	Dyspnea
Hemoptysis	Chest pain
Cough	Sputum

Patient data base (contd.)

Cardiovascular
Palpitation	Blood pressure
Pain	Orthopnia
Murmurs	Cyanosis
Edema	Claudication

Gastrointestinal
Appetite	Pain
Hematemesis	Jaundice
Hernia	Melena/hematochezia/stool color
Constipation	Anal discomfort
Stool shape	Hemorrhoids
Dysphagia	Indigestion
Diarrhea	Abdominal girth
Nausea, vomiting	

Genitourinary
Dysuria	Urine color/hematuria
Nocturia	Hesitancy
Frequency	Urgency
Incontinence	Enuresis

Reproductive
Syphilis, gonorrhea, sores	
Discharge	Intercourse
Sterility	Contraception

(Males)
Epididymitis	Pain
Impotence	Prostate disease

(Females)
Dyspareunia	Menarche
Cycle/duration/amount/menopause/last monthly period	
Last pelvic exam	
Dysmenorrhea	Spotting
Irregularity	
Gravida/para/abortions	

Breasts
Lumps	Pain
Discharge	Self-exam.

Endocrine
Goiter	Glycosuria
Treatment with hormones	
Heat/cold intolerance	

Allergic
Eczema	Asthma
Hay fever	Hives

Bones, muscles, joints
Trauma	Pain
Swelling	Stiffness

Blood-lymphatic
Anemia	Bleeding
Bruising	
Lymph node enlargement	

Neurological
Syncope	Convulsions
Sensation	Coordination
Gait	Paralysis, strength

Psychological
Memory	Mood
Sleep pattern	Stress
Nervousness	
Emotional disturbances	
Drug, alcohol problems	

ASSESSMENT INSTRUMENT 12

I. Rating scale: Interviewing skills (physician's assistant)

II. Competences to be assessed:
History-taking
Communication

III. Specific abilities to be assessed:
1. Ability to establish rapport with patient.
2. Ability to elicit and recognize pertinent information.
3. Ability to summarize and clarify responses.
4. Ability to project sincerity and professional consideration for patient as regards confidentiality.
5. Ability to interpret and report patients' non-verbal behaviour.

IV. Purpose of assessment: formative or summative.
Designed to explore student's mastery of the process of interviewing. Observer not expected to assess the subject of the questioning so much as the ease and style with which it is carried out. Could be used for pre-test, periodic assessment, or end-of-course assessment.

V. Comments:
Scoring is simply "satisfactory", "unsatisfactory", or "cannot rate". Criteria for the first two variables are provided for ten areas of interviewing performance. No evaluation data are available. Has been used in physician's-assistant programme.

VI. Source to contact for further information:
Martha Duhamel
MEDEX Northwest
University of Washington
Seattle, WA
USA

INTERVIEW CRITIQUE SHEET

Directions: Anchor-point criteria are provided for each variable on a continuum from "satisfactory" (S) to "unsatisfactory" (U). Each student should be judged on every variable and a check ( ) placed in the box which indicates the student's performance on the continuum. If you cannot rate a student on a variable, check the right-hand column.

_____

Observer (self or other)

Date_____

SATISFACTORY (S) CRITERIA

1. Opening remarks
Greets patient by name, with appropriate social gestures (handshakes, etc.). Introduces self; explains purpose of interview. Time frame explained, and patient's consent obtained. Sufficient time spent to establish rapport. Attention paid to both comfort and privacy of patient and interviewer.
Comments:

UNSATISFACTORY (U) CRITERIA

Brusque introduction. Insufficient time spent on social amenities. Unclear introduction and explanation of purpose of interview. Insensitive to patient's anxiety or need for comfort and privacy. Authoritarian rather than collaborative role assumed by interviewer.
Comments:

S |__|__|__|__| U

1.

2. Non-verbal communication:
Interviewer demonstrates an interest in what the patient is saying by eye contact, leaning forward, encouraging looks, and nodding (where appropriate).
Comments:

Interviewer looks away from patient; turns back on patient; or stands up prematurely, cutting off patient. Manner and body language reflect lack of interest and concern with patient.
Comments:

S |__|__|__|__| U

2.

3. Questioning skills, types:
Questions are simple and brief. Asks open-ended questions and progresses to focused and closed questions only when specific information necessary.
Comments:

Interviewer consistently asks closed questions, prematurely ending discussion. Asks confusing or compound questions.

Comments:

S |__|__|__|__| U

3.

4. Questioning-summary/clarification:
Summarizes interview content periodically. Asks questions to clarify meaning, and to obtain a fuller understanding of the history.
Comments:

Fails to clarify confusing responses from the patient. Does not summarize; or uses summary only at end of interview.
Comments:

S |__|__|__|__| U

4.

5. Questioning skills, control:
Interviewer is able to let the interview progress spontaneously to obtain the whole story, but redirects it when it becomes irrelevant or fragmented. Uses appropriate reinforcing cues (i.e., eye contact, leaning forward, nodding, smiling, repeating key words and phrases, etc.) or restricting cues (i.e., stops reinforcing cues, directs statements, etc.).
Comments:

Interview is often unfocused, and apparently out of the interviewer's control. Does not use restricting or reinforcing cues; or uses them inappropriately.

Comments:

S |__|__|__|__| U

5.

Cannot rate

INTERVIEW CRITIQUE SHEET (contd)

SATISFACTORY (S) CRITERIA	UNSATISFACTORY (U) CRITERIA	Cannot rate

6. *Listening skills, general:*
Effectively uses silence to draw out patient. Uses active listening techniques, when appropriate, such as restatement, summarizing, and "prodding statements". Uses interpretation when appropriate.
Comments:

Interviewer talks too much; rarely restates what has been said; uses few or no summary or clarifying statements; uses misplaced or inappropriate interpretations.

Comments:

S ☐☐☐☐ U

6.

7. *Listening skills, empathy:*
Demonstrates ability to reflect back empathically to the patient what the patient has said; is sensitive to mood and feelings of the patient.
Comments:

Makes statements that appear to lack empathy or appear hostile or abrasive in the context of the interview; is insensitive to mood and feeling of the patient.
Comments:

S ☐☐☐☐ U

7.

8. *Personal mannerisms:*
Interviewer is relatively free of distracting personal mannerisms during the interview. Facial expressions convey acceptance. Body posture and position are appropriate.

Comments:

Distracting personal mannerisms are present during the interview such as nail-biting, nail-cleaning, hair-pulling, tooth-picking, or slumping in chair. Interviewer seems unaware of these. Facial expression conveys disgust or annoyance. Body posture and position are inappropriate.
Comments:

S ☐☐☐☐ U

8.

9. *Student's observations:*
Student can accurately recall and report observations of the patient's behavioural "physical status" (body posture and care, mood, speech, mannerisms, body position, and movement).
Comments:

Interviewer does not notice and cannot discuss the behavior of the patient.

Comments:

S ☐☐☐☐ U

9.

10. *Expression of personal competence:*
Interviewer's conduct is characterized by consideration and respect; reports facts accurately, including own errors. Respects property of others and the confidence of the patient. Projects an attitude of confidence and ease.
Comments:

Interviewer often inept and unsure, behavior does not convey consideration or respect for the patient or the patient's property. Gossips about the patient. Interviewer falsifies information or defensively avoids accepting responsibility for own behavior.
Comments:

S ☐☐☐☐ U

10.

Additional comments:

Evaluator's overall judgement:
_____ Performance definitely adequate
_____ Performance (tape) should be reviewed by entire staff
_____ Performance definitely inadequate

Further comments:

ASSESSMENT INSTRUMENT 13

I. Rating scale: Physical and mental examination (physician)

II. Competences to be assessed:
Data-gathering
Communication

III. Specific abilities to be assessed:
1. Ability to carry out, interpret, and record correctly physical and mental tests and procedures.
2. Ability to conduct a physical examination, minimizing possible discomfort or embarrassment on the part of the patient.
3. Ability to employ diagnostic instruments correctly.

IV. Purpose of assessment: formative.
Used with medical students in course or interviewing and introduction to clinical medicine.

V. Comments:
No formal evaluation done so far.

VI. Source to contact for further information:
Sandra Lass
Department of Medical Education
University of Southern California School of Medicine
1975 Zonal Ave.
Los Angeles, CA 90033
USA

GENERAL INFORMATION FORM

Student's name _____   Please check one:
Instructor's name _____   _____ Patient interview
Date_____Time _____   _____ Patient physical examination

Type of patient seen (please check one in each column):

_____ ambulatory   _____ male   _____ adult   _____ age of patient
_____ bed-bound   _____ female   _____ child   or informant

General description of patient's illness (please check one):

_____ (1) acute illness (in previously healthy person)
_____ (2) recurring disease with an acute episode
_____ (3) acute multisystem disease
_____ (4) chronic disease (new events, related)
_____ (5) chronic disease (new events, unrelated)
_____ (6) readmission or recently discharged patient (interval history; check-up or follow-up visit)
_____ (7) other: please describe _____

CONDUCT OF THE PHYSICAL EXAMINATION

The form for evaluating the conduct of a physical examination includes nine groups of features to be examined by the student and three other factors relevant to the assessment. The groups of features are listed in the first column and include: general appearance; head and neck; thorax and lungs; heart; abdomen; extremities; rectum; genitalia; and mental status. The lettered areas listed under each of the nine groups of features are to be checked (✓) as the student examines them. The last three columns list the following factors: (1) student-patient relationship, e.g., adequacy of communication and the rapport the student establishes and maintains with the patient; consideration for the patient's physical and psychological comfort; explanation of the procedures of the examination; concern for the patient's modesty and dignity; (2) techniques or modes of examination, e.g., adequacy of inspection, palpation, percussion, and ausculation; appropriateness of the posture or position in which the student places himself and the patient as the examinations of the various regions are conducted (patient sitting up or lying on back, student standing at the foot or at the side of the bed); (3) use of diagnostic instruments, e.g., flashlight, tongue blade, ophthalmoscope, otoscope, stethoscope, reflex hammer, sphygmomanometer. For each of the nine groups of features the student examined, please indicate the extent to which the student demonstrated proficiency in the items listed under each of the three factors. Do this in the following manner:

1. For each of the nine groups of features:
   check (✓) each of the lettered areas that the student examined.
2. For each item listed under each of the three factors:
   write (+) if the student demonstrated *satisfactory* performance,
   write (−) if the student demonstrated *unsatisfactory* performance,
   write (O) if the item listed was *not demonstrated* by the student,
   write (NA) if the item listed was *not applicable* to the situation.
3. For each item in which the student demonstrated *unsatisfactory* performance, please explain the nature of the difficulty or problem in the space provided at the end of the form.

Features examined	Other factors		
(Please check (✓) each lettered feature examined by the student)	(Please indicate (+), (−), (O), or (NA) for each item listed under the three factors)		
	Student-patient relationship	Techniques or modes of examination	Use of diagnostic instruments
1. *General appearance and behavior*			
____ (a) state of consciousness	____ communication; rapport	____ inspection	
____ (b) skin color			
____ (c) gait	____ consideration for comfort	____ patient s position	
____ (d) skin (dry and or dehydrated; moist)	____ explanation of procedures	____ student's position	
____ (e) mood	concern for modesty, dignity		
(f) state of nutrition			

Features examined (Please check (✓) each lettered feature examined by the student)	Other factors (Please indicate (+), (–), (O), or (NA) for each item listed under the three categories)		
	Student-patient relationship	Techniques or modes of examination	Use of diagnostic instruments
2. Head and neck ___(a) head ___(b) eyes ___(c) ears ___(d) nose ___(e) mouth and pharynx ___(f) neck	(Complete only if different from above) ___communication; rapport ___consideration for comfort ___explanation of procedures ___concern for modesty, dignity	___inspection ___palpation ___ausculation ___patient's position ___student's position	___flashlight ___tongue blade ___ophthalmoscope ___otoscope ___stethoscope
3. Thorax and Lungs ___(a) back ___(b) posterior thorax and lungs ___(c) anterior thorax and lungs ___(d) breasts and axillary regions	(Complete only if different from above) ___communication; rapport ___consideration for comfort ___explanation of procedures ___concern for modesty, dignity	___inspection ___palpation ___percussion ___auscultation ___patient's position ___student's position	___stethoscope
4. Heart ___(a) cardiac apical impulse ___(b) cardiac border ___(c) aortic area ___(d) pulmonic area ___(e) mitral area ___(f) tricuspic area	(Complete only if different from above) ___communication; rapport ___consideration for comfort ___explanation of procedures ___concern for modesty, dignity	___inspection ___palpation ___percussion ___auscultation ___patient's position ___student's position	___stethoscope
5. Abdomen ___(a) abdominal wall, intestines ___(b) liver ___(c) spleen ___(d) bladder ___(e) kidneys ___(f) abdominal aorta ___(g) inguinal region	(Complete only if different from above) ___communication; rapport ___consideration for comfort ___explanation of procedures ___concern for modesty, dignity	___inspection ___light palpation ___deep palpation ___bimanual palpation ___percussion ___auscultation ___patient's position ___student's position	___stethoscope
6. Extremities ___(a) skin, nails, muscles, motion ___(b) deep tendon reflexes ___(c) plantar reflex ___(d) pulses ___(e) blood pressure	(Complete only if different from above) ___communication; rapport ___consideration for comfort ___explanation of procedures ___concern for modesty, dignity	___inspection ___palpation ___patient's position ___student's position	___reflex hammer ___sphygmomano-meter

Features examined (Please check (√) each lettered feature examined by the student)	Other factors (Please indicate (+), (−), (O), or (NA) for each item listed under the three categories)		
	Student-patient relationship	Techniques or modes of examination	Use of diagnostic instruments

7.   *Rectum*
(Complete only if different from above)

___(a) perineum
___(b) anus
___(c) perianal area
___(d) pilonidal sinus

___communication;
rapport
___consideration
for comfort
___explanation of
procedures
___concern for
modesty,
dignity

___inspection
___palpation

___patient's position
___student's position

8.   *Genitalia*
(Complete only if different from above)

___*Male*
___(a) pubic hair
___(b) scrotum
___(c) penis
___(d) glans
___(e) penile shaft,
penile urethra
___(f) perineum
___(g) inguinal, femoral
regions

___communication;
rapport
___consideration
for comfort
___explanation of
procedures
___concern for
modesty,
dignity

___inspection
palpation

___patient's position
___student's position

___*Female*
___(a) pubic hair
___(b) labia
___(c) clitoris
___(d) introitus
___(e) urethral orifice
___(f) perineal area
___(g) anus

9   *Mental status*
(Complete only if different from above)

___(a) behavior
___(b) cognition function
___(c) thought content
___(d) perception
___(e) affect and mood

___communication;
rapport
___consideration
for comfort
explanation of
procedures
___concern for
modesty, dignity

___inspection

___patient's position
___student's position

___Using the same scale (+) *satisfactory*, (−) *unsatisfactory*, and (NA) *not applicable*, please indicate your impression of the student's performance throughout the entire physical examination. Do this for each of the items listed below.
  ___organization, sequence of examination
  ___speed of examination
  ___thoroughness of examination
___Please explain the nature of the problem regarding any items in which the student demonstrated *unsatisfactory* performance.
___Please comment on any other factors not included on this form that may have affected the student's conduct of the physical examination. Please include both positive and negative factors.

ASSESSMENT INSTRUMENT 14

I. Check-list: Physical examination (physician's assistant)

II. Competences to be assessed:
Data-gathering
Physical examination

III. Specific abilities to be assessed:
1. Ability to conduct examination expertly and properly.
2. Ability to employ common medical instruments effectively.

IV. Purpose of assessment: summative.
Used as final examination at end of course for physician's assistants. Currently in use to assess extent of knowledge of a physical examination.

V. Comments:
Instrument has not been evaluated and no data are available regarding its validity. Student does not have the instrument as a reference; rater checks off the tasks the student elects to include. Those not done are left blank. A qualitative assessment is elicited as the second part of the instrument.

VI. Source to contact for further information:
Physician Assistant Program
George Washington University Medical Center
Washington, DC
USA

STUDENT EVALUATION FORM
PHYSICIAN'S ASSISTANT PROGRAM

Physical Examination

Student: _____   Instructor: _____

INSTRUCTIONS: Please fill out one form on each student after having directly
observed the student performing a physical. Ask the student to verbally identify
to you each item he observes as he is performing his physical examination.
(Example: I am now observing the symmetry of the head.)

The evaluation form is divided into two sections. The first section is an inclusion-
deletion section to determine which tasks the student included in the physical
examination, regardless of how well or badly he performed these tasks. The second
section evalutes qualitative features of performance. Space is provided for comments at the end of the second section.

I. Physical Examination Inclusions. Check off those tasks which the student
    includes in his examination. If the task is incompletely performed, place an
    (I) in the appropriate space. If the student does not perform the task,
    leave the space blank.

    A. Vital Signs
        Blood pressure determination, both arms   R____ L____
        Radial pulse palpation   R____ L____

    B. Head
        Inspection of head and face
        Palpation of skull, scalp and hair   ____
        Palpation of masseter and temporal muslces (C.N. V Motor) ____
        Assessment of C.N. VII (motor):
            elevate eyebrows, frown, close eyes tightly,
            puff out cheeks, smile   ____

    C. Eyes
        Inspection of upper lids, lower lids, lacrimal ducts R____ L____
            conjunctivae and sclerae
        Assessment of Visual Acuity (C.N.II) (by use of R____ L____
            pocket screener)
        Assessment of extra-ocular movements   R____ L____
            (C.N. III, IV, VI)
        Test for convergence
        Test for pupillary accommodation   ____
        Test visual fields by confrontation (C.N. II) R____ L____
        Test for pupillary reaction to light (direct   R____ L____
            and consensual)
        Test for corneal reflex (C.N. V)   R____ L____
        Performance of funduscopic examination (C.N. II) R____ L____

    D. Ears
        Inspection of external appearance   R____ L____
        Palpation of ear lobes   R____ L____
        Inspection of ear canal and tympanic membrane R____ L____
            by use of otoscope
        Test for gross hearing (C.N. VIII)   R____ L____
        Performance of Weber Test (C.N. VIII)   R____ L____
        Performance of Rinne's Test (C.N. VIII)   R____ L____

    E. Nose
        Inspection of external appearance   R____ L____
        Assessment of nasal patency   R____ L____
        Test sense of smell (C.N. I)   R____ L____
        Inspection of septum, turbinates, and   R____ L____
            nasal mucosa by otoscope
        Palpation or percussion of maxillary sinus   R____ L____
        Palpation or percussion of frontal sinus   R____ L____

F. Mouth and Throat
     Inspection of mouth (lips, teeth, buccal mucosa,
       gums, tongue, hard palate, salivary gland,
       ducts) using tongue blade and flash light   ____
     Inspection of throat (soft palate, uvula,
       tonsillar fossae, phrynx)
     Request that patient phonate during inspection
       of throat (C.N. IX, X)   ____
     Test for gag reflect (C.N. IX, X)   ____
     Request patient to protrude tongue (C.N. XII)   ____

G. Neck
     Inspection of anterior neck   ____
     Request that patient swallow during inspection ____
     Assessment of neck range of motion
       Flexion-extension
       Lateral flextion   ____
       Lateral rotation
     Sternocleidomastoid against resistance (C.N. XI) ____
     Palpation of lymph nodes
       Pre-auricular   R____ L____
       Post-auricular   R____ L____
       Occipital   R____ L____
       Tonsillar   R____ L____
       Submaxillary and Submental   R____ L____
       Superficial cervical   R____ L____
       Posterior cervical chain   R____ L____
       Deep cervical chain   R____ L____
       Supraclavicular   R____ L____
     Palpation of tracheal position   ____
     Palpation of thyroid from posterior approach ____
     Request that patient swallow during thyroid palpation ____

H. Back
     Inspection of spine and skin   ____
     Palpation of:
       Thorax   R____ L____
       Lower back   R____ L____
     Percussion of spine
     Percussion of costovertebral angle   R____ L____

I. Chest-posterior approach - sitting
     Inspection of chest movement on deep inspiration ____
     Palpation of chest movement on deep inspiration ____
     Palpation for tactile fremitus:
       Apices   R____ L____
       Posterior thorax   R____ L____
       Lateral thorax   R____ L____
     Percussion of chest:
       Apices   R____ L____
       Posterior thorax   R____ L____
       Lateral thorax   R____ L____
     Percussion for diaphragmatic excursion   R____ L____
     Auscultation of lung fields:
       Apices   R____ L____
       Posterior thorax   R____ L____
       Lateral thorax   R____ L____

J. Chest-anterior approach - sitting
     Inspection of anterior thorax   R____ L____
     Palpation of anterior thorax   R____ L____
     Palpation for tactile fremitus   R____ L____
     Percussion of anterior thorax   R____ L____
     Auscultation of anterior thorax   R____ L____

K. Breasts and Axillae
     Inspection of breast: Sitting
       Arms at side   R____ L____
       Arms on Hips   R____ L____
       Overhead   R____ L____

P. 3

Palpation of:	Sitting	Supine
Breast	R___ L___	R___ L___
Nipple	R___ L___	R___ L___
Axillary lymph nodes	R___ L___	R___ L___

L. Heart
    Inspection of neck veins   R___ L___
    Inspection of precordium
    Palpation of carotid artery (one at a time)   ___
    Palpation for:
        A. Precordial thrills, etc.   ___
        B. Apical impulse   ___
    Palpation of suprasternal notch   ___
    Percussion of heart borders   ___
    Auscultation at the following points:

	Diaphragm	Bell
Right second interspace adjacent to sternum (aortic area)	___	___
Left second interspace adjacent to sternum (pulmonic area)	___	___
Third left interspace adjacent to sternum (Erb s point)	___	___
Fifth left interspace close to the sternum) (tricuspid area)	___	___
Fifth left interspace just medial to the midclavicular line (mitrial (apical) area)	___	___
Auscultation of carotid arteries	R___	L___

M. Abdomen - Supine
    Inspection of abdomen   ___

Auscultation:		Auscultation
Right upper quadrant		___
Left upper quadrant		___
Right lower quadrant		___
Left lower quadrant		___
Aorta		___
Renal arteries		R___ L___
Femoral arteries		R___ L___

Palpation of abdomen:	Lightly	Deep
Right upper quadrant	___	___
Left upper quadrant	___	___
Right lower quadrant	___	___
Left lower quadrant	___	___
Percussion:		
General abdomen		___
Upper and lower liver borders		___
Gastric air bubble		___
Spleen		___
Bladder		___
Palpation (deep) for:		
Liver (starting low)		___
Spleen		___
Kidneys		R___ L___
Bowels		___
Aorta		___
Femoral artery		R___ L___
Lymph nodes inguinal		R___ L___

N. Extremities
    Inspection of upper extremities

Fingernails		R___ L___
Fingers		R___ L___
Forearm		R___ L___
Upper arm and shoulder		R___ L___
Palpation of:		

	Joints	Muscle Groups
Fingers (Distal interphalangeals)	R___ L___	R___ L___
(Middle interphalangeals)	R___ L___	R___ L___
(Metacarpels)	R___ L___	R___ L___
Wrist	R___ L___	R___ L___
Forearm	R___ L___	R___ L___
Elbow	R___ L___	R___ L___
Upper arm	R___ L___	R___ L___
Shoulder	R___ L___	R___ L___
Clavicle	R___ L___	R___ L___

P. 4

Palpation of:
    Epitrochlear lymph nodes   R____ L____
    Brachial pulse   R____ L____
Assessment of ROM:

		Active
Fingers:	extension	R____ L____
	flexion	R____ L____
	abduction	R____ L____
	adduction	R____ L____
Wrist:	flexion	R____ L____
	extension	R____ L____
Elbow:	flexion	R____ L____
	extension	R____ L____
	supination	R____ L____
	pronation	R____ L____
Neck:	extension	R____ L____
	flexion	R____ L____
	lateral flexion	R____ L____
	lateral rotation	R____ L____
Shoulder:	adduction	R____ L____
	abduction	R____ L____
	internal rotation	R____ L____
	external rotation	R____ L____
Muscle Strength:	fingers	R____ L____
	wrist	R____ L____
	forearm	R____ L____
	upper arm	R____ L____
	shoulder	R____ L____

Extremities Lower (Supine):
Inspection of

Toenails		R____ L____
Toes		R____ L____
Ankle		R____ L____
Lower leg		R____ L____
Knee		R____ L____
Upper leg		R____ L____

Palpation of:

	Joints	Muscle Groups
Toes	R____ L____	R____ L____
Metatarsel heads	R____ L____	R____ L____
Ankle	R____ L____	R____ L____
Lower leg	R____ L____	R____ L____
Knee	R____ L____	R____ L____
Upper leg	R____ L____	R____ L____

Palpation of

Popliteal pulse	R____ L____
Dorsalis pedis pulse	R____ L____
Posterior tibial pulse	R____ L____
Peripheral pitting edema	R____ L____

Assessment of ROM:

		Active
Toes:	flexion	R____ L____
	extension	R____ L____
Ankle:	inversion	R____ L____
	eversion	R____ L____
	dorsiflexion	R____ L____
	plantar flexion	R____ L____
Knee:	flexion	R____ L____
	extension	R____ L____
Hip:	flexion	R____ L____
	abduction	R____ L____
	adduction	R____ L____
	internal rotation	R____ L____
	external rotation	R____ L____

Motor:

	Muscle Strength
Toes	R____ L____
Ankle	R____ L____
Lower leg	R____ L____
Upper Leg	R____ L____
Hip	R____ L____

P. 5

O. Genitalia--Male (If not
    applicable, check here ____.)
    Inspection of penis, scrotum, hair, meatus
    Palpation of:
        Penis and meatus
        Scrotal contents
    Palpation for inguinal hernia   R____ L____

P. Rectal Exam
    Inspection of perianal area
    Palpation for fissures, hemorrhoids, spincter
        tone, prostate, masses
    *Occult blood test (This is a lab procedure
        but should be done at this time.)

O. Neurological
    Mental status:
        Orientation to person, place, time
        Recent and remote memory
        Reasoning (proverbs)
        Cerebration (serial 7's, etc.)
    Cerebellar function:
        Inspection of gait and posture   R____ L____
        Rapid alternating movements   R____ L____
        Finger-to-nose test   R____ L____
        Romberg test   R____ L____
    Sensation: Upper Extremity   Lower Extremity
        Sharp/dull   R____ L____   R____ L____
        Light touch   R____ L____   R____ L____
        Vibration   R____ L____   R____ L____
        Temperature   R____ L____   R____ L____
    Deep Tendon Reflex:
        Biceps   R____ L____
        Triceps   R____ L____
        Brachioradialis   R____ L____
        Patellar   R____ L____
        Achilles   R____ L____
        Plantar   R____ L____
                                      Upper Extremity
    Proprioception   R____ L____
    (position sense)
    Stereognosis   R____ L____
    (coin/key recognition)

II. Qualitative Assessment of Performance   YES   NO

    A. Student positions the patient properly for examination ____   ____
    B. Student positions himself properly in relation to the   ____   ____
            patient during examination
    C. Student drapes the patient properly during examination ____   ____
    D. Student exposes areas properly for examination   ____   ____
    E. Student uses a systematic approach to the total exam-   ____   ____
            ination and to regional examination
    F. Performs palpation technique as taught for all areas:
            abd   ____   ____
            muscle groups   ____   ____
    G. Performs percussion as taught for all areas   ____   ____
    H. Performs auscultation technique as taught   ____   ____
    I. Uses the following instruments as taught:
            Sphygmomanometer   ____   ____
            Stethoscope   ____   ____
            Ophthalmoscope   ____   ____
            Otoscope   ____   ____
            Reflex hammer   ____   ____

P. 6

Additional Comments on Student Performance:

_____

_____

_____

_____

_____

_____

_____

_____

OVERALL RATING:

Outstanding	Very Good	Average	Below Average	Marginal or Unacceptable
5	4	3	2	1

PERFORMANCE OF SPECIFIC TASKS

Type of instrument	Task	Category of personnel	Reference number	Page
Check-list	Specific clinical skills	Nurse	15	122
Check-list and rating scale	Cardiovascular examination	Physician	16	134
Rating scale	Physical therapy	Physical therapy assistant	17	141
Rating scale	Anaesthetic processes	Nurse anaesthetist	18	144
Rating scale	Surgical nursing	Nurse	19	147
Check-list	Physical examination (heart, lungs, abdomen)	Physician's assistant	20	150
Rating scale	Nursing activities	Nurse	21	153
Check-list	Paediatric cardiac catheterization	Physician	22	159
Rating scale	Respiratory therapy	Respiratory therapist	23	162
Check-list	Radiation oncology	Radiation therapist	24	164
Rating scale	Patient education	Physician's assistant	25	166
Check-list	Dental hygiene procedures	Dental hygienist	26	168
Check-list	Maternity care	Traditional birth attendant	27	171

ASSESSMENT INSTRUMENT 15

I. Check-list: Specific clinical skills (nurse)

II. Competences to be assessed: clinical skills required to perform the following activities

1. Taking temperature
   Counting pulse
   Counting respirations
   Taking blood pressure
2. Bedmaking
   Positioning patient
3. Bathing patient
   Care of pressure areas
   Mouth care
   Hair care
4. Oxygen administration
   —by mask
   —by nasal catheter
   —by nasal prongs
5. Changing a dressing
   Removing sutures
   Removing clips
   Shortening/removing drains
6. Establishing/maintaining an airway
   Insertion of an artificial airway
7. Insertion of a nasogastric tube
   Removal of a nasogastric tube

8. Feeding via a nasogastric tube
   Irrigation of a nasogastric tube
9. Medication, by mouth
   —by injection (intramuscular, hypodermic)
   —by injection (intravenous)
10. Medication, ears
    —eyes
    —nose
11. Catheterization
    —indwelling
    Bladder irrigation
12. Intermittent positive pressure therapy
    Cough and deep breathing exercises
13. Tracheostome care
    —suctioning
    —change of tube

III. Specific abilities to be assesed:
1. Ability to perform specified nursing care techniques and procedures.
2. Ability to adapt procedures to individual patient tolerance and condition.
3. Ability to carry out procedures deftly, with a minimum of discomfort or embarrassment on the part of the patient.

IV. Purpose of assessment: Summative.
   Used to assess performance in each of the tested areas of patient care. Each separate test result is made available at the time, and a composite score forms the clinical achievement component of the requirements of registration as a trained nurse.

V. Comments:
   Reliability and validity studies have been made, and statistical data
   are available.

VI. Source to contact for further information:
   Ruth White
   University of New South Wales
   Tertiary Education Research Centre
   Sydney, N.S.W.
   Australia

CLINICAL SKILLS ASSESSMENT TOOLS
Advice to student and observer

The observer must ensure that, in addition to the activities on the test form, the student also performs the following activities for each test:

Activities common to all tests:
A. Washes hands both before and after the procedure.
B. Organizes requirements and equipment before commencing the test.
C. Cleans away the equipment following the procedure.
D. Reports and records observations and activities.

Protection of the patient and the student:
The assessment must cease if, in the judgment of the observer:
1. The patient is under any threat of physical, emotional, or environmental danger.
2. The student is an unprepared candidate, i.e.,
   (a) has not performed common activities A and/or B
   (b) shows evidence of insufficient prior learning, or
   (c) shows extreme nervousness.

CLINICAL SKILLS ASSESSMENT TOOL 1

Activities:
( )   Temperature   1–4
( )   Pulse   5–7
( )   Respirations   8–10
( )   Blood pressure   11–16

Patient situation:

	Observed	Not observed
Temperature:		
1. Ensures the thermometer is ready for use. _____	( )	( )
2. Positions the thermometer in axilla, in rectum, or under the tongue (in a mouth free from temperature-altering substances at least 5 minutes) as dictated by patient condition, age, and/or hospital policy. _____	( )	( )
3. Removes the thermometer after a minimum of 2 minutes. _____	( )	( )
4. Reads the thermometer within ± 0.1° C. _____	( )	( )
Pulse:		
5. Counts the pulse for no less than 30 seconds for regular pulse, 60 seconds for irregular pulse. _____	( )	( )
6. States rhythm and rate of the pulse. _____	( )	( )
7. States the rate within accuracy of ± 4. _____	( )	( )
Respirations:		
8. Ensures visibility of chest movement. _____	( )	( )
9. Counts the number of respirations for no less than 30 seconds if normal, 60 seconds if abnormal. _____	( )	( )
10. States the rate and pattern of respirations. _____	( )	( )
Blood pressure:		
11. Establishes patient's average systolic pressure by referring to blood pressure chart or using radial palpation method. _____	( )	( )
12. Applies the cuff placing the balloon over the area of the brachial artery. __	( )	( )
13. Places stethoscope over the antecubital fossa. _____	( )	( )
14. Inflates the cuff 10–20 mm above pre-estimated systolic pressure. _____	( )	( )
15. Deflates the cuff slowly. _____	( )	( )
16. Reads the mercury level at the first sound heard, and at the change in sound or at the last sound heard within an accuracy of ± 4 mm. _____	( )	( )

Behaviour guides:	Yes	No	N/A[1]
i. Approaches the patient with confidence and courtesy. _____	( )	( )	( )
ii. Gives a relevant explanation in ways the patient can understand. ____	( )	( )	( )
iii. Orients the patient to possible discomfort and to his role during the procedure. _____	( )	( )	( )
iv. Anticipates patient's embarrassment and protects privacy. _____	( )	( )	( )
v. Makes allowances for individual concern about the observations. ____	( )	( )	( )
vi. Shows patience. _____	( )	( )	( )
vii. Notices cues indicating patient's discomfort and attempts to alleviate it.	( )	( )	( )
viii. Paces the procedure appropriately to tolerance and/or condition of patient. _____	( )	( )	( )
ix. Focuses attention on the procedure to the extent that readiness to respond to other events is limited. _____	( )	( )	( )
x. Indicates awareness of responsibility to the patient following the procedure. _____	( )	( )	( )

---

[1]N/A = not applicable

CLINICAL SKILLS ASSESSMENT TOOL 2

Activities:
( ) Bedmaking   1–6
( ) Positioning   7–10

Patient situation:

	Observed	*Not observed*
Bedmaking:		
1. Untucks and lifts clear of self each individual article of linen from bed. ___	( )	( )
2. Places linen on bed without flourishing. ___	( )	( )
3. Ensures bottom sheet is tucked in tightly, removing wrinkles. ___	( )	( )
4. Ensures adequate tuck-in at top of bed. ___	( )	( )
5. Positions top linen to prevent pressure. ___	( )	( )
6. Ensures top linen will provide enough cover. ___	( )	( )
Positioning:		
7. Assembles adequate means of assistance. ___	( )	( )
8. Instructs patient about his role in the move. ___	( )	( )
9. Re-positions patient with maximal support and minimal discomfort. _	( )	( )
10. Re-establishes patient's body alignment, using whatever supportive aids required. ___	( )	( )

	Yes	*No*	*N/A*[1]
Behaviour guides:			
i. Approaches the patient with confidence and courtesy. ___	( )	( )	( )
ii. Gives a relevant explanation in ways the patient can understand. ___	( )	( )	( )
iii. Orients the patient to possible discomfort and to his role during the procedure. ___	( )	( )	( )
iv. Anticipates patient's embarrassment and protects privacy. ___	( )	( )	( )
v. Makes allowances for individual differences in fear of movement and tolerance of pain. ___	( )	( )	( )
vi. Shows patience. ___	( )	( )	( )
vii. Notices cues indicating patient's discomfort and attempts to alleviate it.	( )	( )	( )
viii. Paces the procedure appropriately to tolerance and/or condition of patient. ___	( )	( )	( )
ix. Focuses attention on the procedure to the extent that readiness to respond to other events is limited. ___	( )	( )	( )
x. Indicates awarensss of responsibility to the patient following the procedure. ___	( )	( )	( )

[1] *N A* = not applicable

CLINICAL SKILLS ASSESSMENT TOOL 3

Activities:
( ) Bathing   1–9
( ) Care of pressure areas   1, 10–11
( ) Mouth care   12
( ) Hair care, women   13
    —men   13–14

Patient situation.

	Observed	*Not observed*
General:		
1. Protects privacy throughout the procedure. ___	( )	( )
2. Provides appropriate change of clean, dry attire. ___	( )	( )
Bathing a patient in bed:		
3. Selects temperature of water comfortable to the patient. ___	( )	( )
4. Changes the water as required (minimum of once). ___	( )	( )
5. Removes linen, pillows, and equipment that could hamper bathing. ___	( )	( )
6. Keeps patient adequately covered. ___	( )	( )
7. Washes all areas that are unable to be washed by patient. ___	( )	( )
8. Rinses all areas that are unable to be rinsed by patient. ___	( )	( )
9. Dries all areas that are unable to be dried by patient. ___	( )	( )
Pressure area care:		
10. Massages those areas of potential skin breakdown. ___	( )	( )
11. Minimizes pressure on bony prominences. ___	( )	( )
Mouth care:		
12. Provides/uses (if patient unable) utensils to ensure mouth is free of debris	( )	( )
Hair care.		
13. Ensures hair is kempt. ___	( )	( )
14. Ensures shave (for men) is done, unless contraindicated. ___	( )	( )

CLINICAL SKILLS ASSESSMENT TOOL 3 (*contd.*)

Behaviour guides:	Yes	No	N/A[1]
i. Approaches the patient with confidence and courtesy. _____	( )	( )	( )
ii. Gives a relevant explanation in ways the patient can understand. ___	( )	( )	( )
iii. Orients the patient to possible discomfort and to his role during the procedure. _____	( )	( )	( )
iv. Anticipates patient's embarrassment and protects privacy.. _____	( )	( )	( )
v. Makes allowances for individual differences in needs for communication and responds accordingly. _____	( )	( )	( )
vi. Shows patience. _____	( )	( )	( )
vii. Notices cues indicating patient's discomfort and attempts to alleviate it.	( )	( )	( )
viii. Paces the procedure appropriately to tolerance and/or condition of patient. _____	( )	( )	( )
ix. Focuses attention on the procedure to the extent that readiness to respond to other events is limited. _____	( )	( )	( )
x. Indicates awareness of responsibility to the patient following the procedure. _____	( )	( )	( )

[1]N/A = not applicable

CLINICAL SKILLS ASSESSMENT TOOL 4

Activities:
( )   Administration of oxygen by mask   1–5, 10–11
( )   — by nasal catheter   1–3, 6–8, 10–11
( )   — by nasal prongs   1–3, 9–11

Patient situation:

Oxygen administration:	Observed	Not observed
1. Selects prescribed mode of administration. _____	( )	( )
2. Ensures fluid is at specified level in humidification apparatus. _____	( )	( )
3. Ensures "No smoking" regulations are observed by instructing patient and/or erecting signs. _____	( )	( )
Mask:		
4. Selects mask with reference to patient's facial size/doctor's orders. ___	( )	( )
5. Places mask on patient's face ensuring snug fit around nose and mouth.	( )	( )
Nasal catheter:		
6. Measures length for insertion from tip of patient's nose to lobe of ear.__	( )	( )
7. Lubricates tip of catheter with water-soluble lubricant._____	( )	( )
8. Inserts catheter gently into nares to premeasured distance. _____	( )	( )
Nasal prongs (spectacles):		
9. Inserts prongs inside nares. _____	( )	( )
10. Secures oxygen administration set to prevent dislodgement._____	( )	( )
11. Adjusts humidified oxygen to 3–4 l/min unless otherwise ordered. _____	( )	( )

Behaviour guides:	Yes	No	N/A[1]
i. Approaches the patient with confidence and courtesy. _____	( )	( )	( )
ii. Gives a relevant explanation in ways the patient can understand. ___	( )	( )	( )
iii. Orients the patient to possible discomfort and to his role during the procedure. _____	( )	( )	( )
iv. Anticipates patient's embarrassment and protects privacy. _____	( )	( )	( )
v. Responds to individual differences in fear of symptoms and tolerance of treatment. _____	( )	( )	( )
vi. Shows patience. _____	( )	( )	( )
vii. Notices cues indicating patient's discomfort and attempts to alleviate it.	( )	( )	( )
viii. Paces the procedure appropriately to tolerance and/or condition of patient. _____	( )	( )	( )
ix. Focuses attention on the procedure to the extent that readiness to respond to other events is limited. _____	( )	( )	( )
x. Indicates awareness of responsibility to the patient following the procedure. _____	( )	( )	( )

[1]N/A = not applicable

CLINICAL SKILLS ASSESSMENT TOOL 5

Activities:

( )	Changing dressing	1–8
( )	Removal of sutures	1–4, 9–11
( )	Removal of clips	1–4, 9, 12–14
( )	Shortening drains	1–4, 9, 15–19

Patient situation:

	Observed	Not observed
General:		
1. Opens sterile container without touching contents._____	( )	( )
2. Adds only sterile articles and solutions to sterile field. _____	( )	( )
3. Handles sterile articles with sterile articles. _____	( )	( )
4. Discards contaminated articles immediately into suitable receptacle. ___	( )	( )
Dressing change:		
5. Removes and discards dressing into a suitable receptacle._____	( )	( )
6. Swabs wound in one direction, using each swab once._____	( )	( )
7. Applies and secures sterile dressing. _____	( )	( )
8. Describes the condition of the wound. _____	( )	( )
Removal of sutures:		
9. Removes debris from insertion site._____	( )	( )
10. Cuts sutures close to the skin. _____	( )	( )
11. Pulls the shortest end of the suture through wound. _____	( )	( )
Removal of clips:		
12. Selects appropriate clip remover. _____	( )	( )
13. Eases clip from wound minimizing patient discomfort. _____	( )	( )
14. Cleanses wound (see 6). _____	( )	( )
Shortening/removal of drains:		
15. Withdraws drain completely or to prescribed length. _____	( )	( )
16. Secures sterile safety pin through drain at skin surface. _____	( )	( )
17. Cuts and discards excess drain. _____	( )	( )
18. Cleanses stab wound (see 6). _____	( )	( )
19. Applies and secures sterile dressing. _____	( )	( )

Behaviour guides:	Yes	No	N/A[1]
i. Approaches the patient with confidence and courtesy. _____	( )	( )	( )
ii. Gives a relevant explanation in ways the patient can understand. ___	( )	( )	( )
iii. Orients the patient to possible discomfort and to his role during the procedure._____	( )	( )	( )
iv. Anticipates patient's embarrassment and protects privacy._____	( )	( )	( )
v. Makes allowances for individual differences in fear of treatment and tolerance of pain._____	( )	( )	( )
vi. Shows patience. _____	( )	( )	( )
vii. Notices cues indicating patient's discomfort and attempts to alleviate it.	( )	( )	( )
viii. Paces the procedure appropriately to tolerance and/or condition of patient. _____	( )	( )	( )
ix. Focuses attention on the procedure to the extent that readiness to respond to other events is limited. _____	( )	( )	( )
x. Indicates awareness of responsibility to the patient following the procedure._____	( )	( )	( )

[1]N/A = not applicable

CLINICAL SKILLS ASSESSMENT TOOL 6

Activities:

( )	Establishing and maintaining a patent airway	1–4
( )	Inserting artificial airway	5–10

Patient situation:

	Observed	Not observed
Establishing and maintaining a patent airway:		
1. Ensures adequate visibility of the chest._____	( )	( )
2. Checks that the mouth is free of foreign bodies. _____	( )	( )
3. Hyperextends the patient's head, supporting his neck. _____	( )	( )
4. Elevates the jaw. _____	( )	( )
Insertion of an artificial airway:		
5. Checks that the mouth is free of foreign bodies. _____	( )	( )
6. Hyperextends the patient's head, supporting his neck. _____	( )	( )
7. Introduces the airway, over the tongue in an "inverted S" position. _____	( )	( )

CLINICAL SKILLS ASSESSMENT TOOL 6 (contd.)

8. Rotates the airway to the correct position._____ ( )   ( )
9. Completes insertion of the airway to the phalange._____ ( )   ( )
10. Elevates the jaw. _____ ( )   ( )

Behaviour guides:	Yes	No	N/A[1]
i. Approaches the patient with confidence and courtesy. _____	( )	( )	( )
ii. Gives a relevant explanation in ways the patient can understand. ___	( )	( )	( )
iii. Orients the patient to possible discomfort and to his role during the procedure. _____	( )	( )	( )
iv. Anticipates patient's embarrassment and protects privacy._____	( )	( )	( )
v. Makes allowances for individual differences in fear of symptoms and outcome of present situation. _____	( )	( )	( )
vi. Shows patience. _____	( )	( )	( )
vii. Notices cues indicating patient's discomfort and attempts to alleviate it.	( )	( )	( )
vi. Paces the procedure appropriately to patient tolerance and/or condition of the patient. _____	( )	( )	( )
ix. Focuses attention on the procedure to the extent that readiness to respond to other events is limited. _____	( )	( )	( )
x. Indicates awareness of responsibility to the patient following the procedure. _____	( )	( )	( )

[1]N/A = not applicable

CLINICAL SKILLS ASSESSMENT TOOL 7

Activities:
( )   Insertion of nasogastric tube   1–9
( )   Removal of nasogastric tubes   10–13

Patient situation:

Insertion:	Observed	Not observed
1. Selects nasogastric tube according to order and/or patient size. _____	( )	( )
2. Positions patient in upright or lateral position. _____	( )	( )
3. Measures from tip of patient's nose to ear and to xiphisternum to determine insertion length. _____	( )	( )
4. Lubricates end of tube with water-soluble lubricant. _____	( )	( )
5. Instructs patient to swallow frequently as the tube is being passed. ____	( )	( )
6. Introduces the tube via the nares with smooth motion. _____	( )	( )
7. Advances tube to premeasured distance if no respiratory distress. ____	( )	( )
8. Determines correct position of tube by: _____	( )	( )
(a) aspirating gastric contents and testing pH to confirm acidity, or		
(b) placing free end of the tube under water to determine the absence of bubbles as the patient exhales, or		
(c) some other hospital-accepted method.		
9. Secures tube. _____	( )	( )
Removal:		
10. Untapes the tube._____	( )	( )
11. Occludes the lumen of the tube. _____	( )	( )
12. Instructs the patient to exhale as the tube is removed. _____	( )	( )
13. Cleanses nares following removal of tube._____	( )	( )

Behaviour guides:	Yes	No	N/A[1]
i. Approaches the patient with confidence and courtesy. _____	( )	( )	( )
ii. Gives a relevant explanation in ways the patient can understand. ___	( )	( )	( )
iii. Orients the patient to possible discomfort and to his role during the procedure. _____	( )	( )	( )
iv. Anticipates patient's embarrassment and protects privacy._____	( )	( )	( )
v. Makes allowances for individual differences in fear of treatment and tolerance of pain._____	( )	( )	( )
vi. Shows patience. _____	( )	( )	( )
vii. Notices cues indicating patient's discomfort and attempts to alleviate it.	( )	( )	( )
viii. Paces the procedure appropriately to tolerance and/or condition of patient. _____	( )	( )	( )
ix. Focuses attention on the procedure to the extent that readiness to respond to other events is limited. _____	( )	( )	( )
x. Indicates awareness of responsibility to the patient following the procedure. _____	( )	( )	( )

[1]N/A = not applicable

CLINICAL SKILLS ASSESSMENT TOOL 8

Activities:
( )   Feeding via a nasogastric tube   1–5
( )   Irrigation of a nasogastric tube   1–4, 6–8
Patient situation:

Feeding:

	Observed	Not observed
1. Ensures upright position of patient unless contraindicated. _____	( )	( )
2. Ensures tube is correctly positioned. _____	( )	( )
3. Checks that prescribed fluid is at approximately normal body temperature.	( )	( )
4. Introduces ordered amount of fluid through tube. _____	( )	( )
5. Inserts minimum of 10 ml of water following feed unless otherwise ordered.	( )	( )

Irrigation:

	Observed	Not observed
6. Instills and aspirates fluid, repeating until return is clear. _____	( )	( )
7. Compresses the tube each time syringe is removed. _____	( )	( )
8. Measures amount of fluid on both instillation and removal. _____	( )	( )

Behaviour guides:	Yes	No	N/A[1]
i. Approaches the patient with confidence and courtesy. _____	( )	( )	( )
ii. Gives a relevant explanation in ways the patient can understand. ___	( )	( )	( )
iii. Orients the patient to possible discomfort and to his role during the procedure. _____	( )	( )	( )
iv. Anticipates patient's embarrassment and protects privacy. _____	( )	( )	( )
v. Makes allowances for individual differences in tolerance of treatment.	( )	( )	( )
vi. Shows patience. _____	( )	( )	( )
vii. Notices cues indicating patient's discomfort and attempts to alleviate it.	( )	( )	( )
viii. Paces the procedure appropriately to tolerance and/or condition, of patient. _____	( )	( )	( )
ix. Focuses attention on the procedure to the extent that readiness to respond to other events is limited. _____	( )	( )	( )
x. Indicates awareness of responsibility to the patient following the procedure. _____	( )	( )	( )

[1]*N/A* = not applicable

CLINICAL SKILLS ASSESSMENT TOOL 9

Activities:
( )   Medication by mouth   1–4, 5–6
( )   — by injection (intramuscular, hypodermic)   1–4, 7–12
( )   — by injection (intravenous)   1–4, 7–9, 13–15
Patient situation:

General:

	Observed	Not observed
1. Checks medicament as required by law and/or policy. _____	( )	( )
2. Measures the ordered dose. _____	( )	( )
3. Obtains as unmistakable identification as possible. _____	( )	( )
4. Administers by prescribed route. _____	( )	( )

Oral

5. Provides aid in swallowing. _____	( )	( )
6. Remains with the patient until the medicament is swallowed. _____	( )	( )

By injection (intramuscular, hypodermic):

7. Assembles sterile needle and syringe of appropriate gauge and capacity. ___	( )	( )
8. Aspirates the sterile medicament into syringe. _____	( )	( )
9. Prepares appropriate site. _____	( )	( )
10. Inserts sterile needle at an angle of 45° for hypodermic, 90° for intramuscular injection _____	( )	( )
11. Withdraws plunger (removes needle if blood appears). _____	( )	( )
12. Injects the total dose. _____	( )	( )

By injection (intravenous):

13. Ensures patency of intravenous cannula. _____	( )	( )
14. Ensures that no pressure or kinking is present to impede flow of fluid for injection. _____	( )	( )
15. Injects total dose of fluid over safe period of time. _____	( )	( )

CLINICAL SKILLS ASSESSMENT TOOL 9 (contd.)

Behaviour guides:	Yes	No	N/A[1]
i. Approaches the patient with confidence and courtesy. _____	( )	( )	( )
ii. Gives a relevant explanation in ways the patient can understand. ___	( )	( )	( )
iii. Orients the patient to possible discomfort and to his role during the procedure. _____	( )	( )	( )
iv. Anticipates patient's embarrassment and protects privacy._____	( )	( )	( )
v. Makes allowances for individual differences in fear of treatment and tolerance of pain._____	( )	( )	( )
vi. Shows patience. _____	( )	( )	( )
vii. Notices cues indicating patient's discomfort and attempts to alleviate it.	( )	( )	( )
viii. Paces the procedure appropriately to tolerance and/or condition of patient. _____	( )	( )	( )
ix. Focuses attention on the procedure to the extent that readiness to respond to other events is limited. _____	( )	( )	( )
x. Indicates awareness of responsibility to the patient following the procedure. _____	( )	( )	( )

[1]N/A = not applicable

CLINICAL SKILLS ASSESSMENT TOOL 10

( )   Medication, ears   1–4, 5–9
( )   —eyes   1–4, 10–15
( )   —nose   1–4, 16–18

Patient situation:

General:

	Observed	Not observed
1. Checks medicament as required by law and/or policy. _____	( )	( )
2. Measures the ordered dose. _____	( )	( )
3. Obtains unmistakable identification of patient. _____	( )	( )
4. Administers by prescribed route. _____	( )	( )

Ear drops:

	Observed	Not observed
5. Positions the patient upright with head tilted to one side or in lateral position with affected ear up. _____	( )	( )
6. Draws pinna upwards and backwards (down and back for children). ___	( )	( )
7. Directs dropper towards posterior wall of aural canal. _____	( )	( )
8. Instils drops. _____	( )	( )
9. Asks patient to maintain this position for 10–15 minutes. _____	( )	( )

Eye drops and ointments:

	Observed	Not observed
10. Positions patient with head tilted back. _____	( )	( )
11. Pulls down lower eyelid, directing pressure to malar bone _____	( )	( )
12. Asks patient to look up. _____	( )	( )
13. Instils medicament from 1.5–2 cm approx., avoiding direct fall into cornea.	( )	( )
14. Asks patient to close eye(s). _____	( )	( )
15. Wipes away excess medicament. _____	( )	( )

Nasal drops:

	Observed	Not observed
16. Positions patient with head tilted back. _____	( )	( )
17. Asks patient to breathe through mouth. _____	( )	( )
18. Introduces dropper approx. 1 cm into nostril and instils drops slowly. ___	( )	( )

Behaviour guides:	Yes	No	N/A[1]
i. Approaches the patient with confidence and courtesy. _____	( )	( )	( )
ii. Gives a relevant explanation in ways the patient can understand. ___	( )	( )	( )
iii. Orients the patient to possible discomfort and to his role during the procedure. _____	( )	( )	( )
iv. Anticipates patient's embarrassment and protects privacy. _____	( )	( )	( )
v. Makes allowances for individual differences in fear of treatment and tolerance of pain._____	( )	( )	( )
vi. Shows patience. _____	( )	( )	( )
vii. Notices cues indicating patient's discomfort and attempts to alleviate it.	( )		
viii. Paces the procedure appropriately to tolerance and/or condition of patient. _____	( )	( )	( )
ix. Focuses attention on the procedure to the extent that readiness to respond to other events is limited. _____	( )	( )	( )
x. Indicates awareness of responsibility to the patient following the procedure. _____	( )	( )	( )

[1]N/A = not applicable

CLINICAL SKILLS ASSESSMENT TOOL 11

Activities:

( )	Catheterization	1–9, 13
( )	—indwelling	1–13
( )	Bladder irrigation	1–4, 14–16

Patient situation:

General:

	Observed	Not observed
1. Opens sterile containers without touching contents. _____	( )	( )
2. Adds only sterile articles and solutions to the sterile field. _____	( )	( )
3. Handles sterile articles with sterile articles. _____	( )	( )
4. Discards contaminated articles immediately. _____	( )	( )

Catheterization:

	Observed	Not observed
5. Selects appropriate-sized catheter. _____	( )	( )
6. Lubricates catheter with sterile water-soluble lubricant (anaesthetic lubricant for men). _____	( )	( )
7. Uses sterile catheter for each catheterization attempt. _____	( )	( )
8. Cleanses labia majora, minora then around urinary meatus (glans penis—male). _____	( )	( )
9. Inserts a sterile catheter without force into urethra, approximately 3 in (5.75 cm) for adult female, 7½ in (17.5 cm) for adult male. _____	( )	( )
10. Inflates catheter balloon with no more than stated amount of sterile fluid.	( )	( )
11. Attaches sterile connector to the catheter. _____	( )	( )
12. Takes steps to avoid traction on the catheter. _____	( )	( )
13. Ensures that collection of urine takes place below bladder level. _____	( )	( )

Bladder irrigation:

	Observed	Not observed
14. Selects correct amount of sterile solution as ordered. _____	( )	( )
15. Instils sterile fluid through catheter without the use of force. _____	( )	( )
16. Collects outflow under gravity drainage, into sterile container. _____	( )	( )

Behaviour guides:	Yes	No	N/A
i. Approaches the patient with confidence and courtesy. _____	( )	( )	( )
ii. Gives a relevant explanation in ways the patient can understand. ___	( )	( )	( )
iii. Orients the patient to possible discomfort and to his role during the procedure. _____	( )	( )	( )
iv. Anticipates patient's embarrassment and protects privacy. _____	( )	( )	( )
v. Makes allowances for individual differences in fear of treatment and tolerance of pain. _____	( )	( )	( )
vi. Shows patience. _____	( )	( )	( )
vii. Notices cues indicating patient's discomfort and attempts to alleviate it.	( )	( )	( )
viii. Paces the procedure appropriately to tolerance and or condition of patient. _____	( )	( )	( )
ix. Focuses attention on the procedure to the extent that readiness to respond to other events is limited. _____	( )	( )	( )
x. Indicates awareness of responsibility to the patient following the procedure. _____	( )	( )	( )

[1]N/A = not applicable

CLINICAL SKILLS ASSESSMENT TOOL 12

Activities:
(   ) Intermittent positive pressure therapy   1–7
(   ) Coughing and deep breathing   8–10
Patient situation:

Intermittent positive pressure therapy:	*Observed*	*Not observed*
1. Describes to observer the pattern and rate of the patient's respiration prior to treatment. _____	( )	( )
2. Ensures adequate supply of pressured oxygen or air. _____	( )	( )
3. Adjusts controls to 10–15 cm H_2O unless otherwise ordered. _____	( )	( )
4. Inserts into nebulizer correct amount of fluid as ordered. _____	( )	( )
5. Attaches patient-specific tubing to the correct outlets. _____	( )	( )
6. Ensures patient is using the machine correctly. _____	( )	( )
7. Ceases treatment after therapeutic length of time. _____	( )	( )

Chest physiotherapy—coughing and deep breathing:

	Observed	*Not observed*
8. Places "sputum" receptacle within reach of patient. _____	( )	( )
9. Positions patient so as best to mobilize secretions while allowing for maximum chest expansion. _____	( )	( )
10. Encourages and/or assists patient during coughing and deep breathing. _	( )	( )

Behaviour guides:	*Yes*	*No*	*N/A*[1]
i. Approaches the patient with confidence and courtesy. _____	( )	( )	( )
ii. Gives a relevant explanation in ways the patient can understand. ___	( )	( )	( )
iii. Orients the patient to possible discomfort and to his role during the procedure. _____	( )	( )	( )
iv. Anticipates patient's embarrassment and protects privacy. _____	( )	( )	( )
v. Makes allowances for individual differences in patient's attitudes towards treatment and need for guidance. _____	( )	( )	( )
vi. Shows patience. _____	( )	( )	( )
vii. Notices cues indicating patient's discomfort and attempts to alleviate it.	( )	( )	( )
viii. Paces the procedure appropriately to tolerance and/or condition of patient. _____	( )	( )	( )
ix. Focuses attention on the procedure to the extent that readiness to respond to other events is limited. _____	( )	( )	( )
x. Indicates awareness of responsibility to the patient following the procedure. _____	( )	( )	( )

_____
[1] *N/A* = not applicable

CLINICAL SKILLS ASSESSMENT TOOL 13

Activities:

( )	Tracheostome care	1–8
( )	—suctioning	1–4, 9–15
( )	—change of tube, cuffed	1–7, 16–25
	uncuffed	1–7, 16–17, 19–23, 25

Patient situation:

	Observed	*Not observed*
General:		
1. Opens sterile containers without touching contents. _____	( )	( )
2. Adds only sterile articles and solutions to sterile field. _____	( )	( )
3. Handles sterile articles with sterile articles _____	( )	( )
4. Discards contaminated articles immediately. _____	( )	( )
Tracheostome care:		
5. Removes previous dressing _____	( )	( )
6. Cleanses and dries tracheostome until skin is free of debris. _____	( )	( )
7. Reapplies sterile plain gauze dressing. _____	( )	( )
8. Ties the tape in a knot allowing "give" of one finger. _____	( )	( )
Suctioning:		
9. Suctions nasopharynx and oropharynx, as required _____	( )	( )
10. Uses a sterile catheter for each suctioning. _____	( )	( )
11. Inserts a catheter approx. 20–30 cm gently without suction being applied.	( )	( )
12. Applies suction while removing the catheter in a rotating continuous upward motion. _____	( )	( )
13. Performs 11 and 12 in no more than 10 seconds. _____	( )	( )
14. Suctions tracheostome as completely as possible as determined by patient's condition. _____	( )	( )
15. Discards catheter after use. _____	( )	( )
Change of tube:		
16. Ensures suction apparatus is ready for use. _____	( )	( )
17. Ensures sterile tracheostomy dilator is at the bedside. _____	( )	( )
18. Deflates cuff. _____	( )	( )
19. Releases ties. _____	( )	( )
20. Withdraws tracheostomy tube as patient exhales. _____	( )	( )
21. Suctions as required. _____	( )	( )
22. Cleanses and dries tracheostome until skin is free of debris. _____	( )	( )
23. Inserts sterile tracheostomy tube into stomal opening. _____	( )	( )
24. Inflates cuff just to the point of absence of air leak. _____	( )	( )
25. Ties the tape in a knot allowing "give" of one finger. _____	( )	( )

Behaviour guides:	*Yes*	*No*	*N/A*[1]
i. Approaches the patient with confidence and courtesy. _____	( )	( )	( )
ii. Gives a relevant explanation in ways the patient can understand _____	( )	( )	( )
iii. Orients the patient to possible discomfort and to his role during the procedure. _____	( )	( )	( )
iv. Anticipates patient's embarrassment and protects privacy. _____	( )	( )	( )
v. Makes allowances for individual differences in fear of treatment and tolerance of pain. _____	( )	( )	( )
vi. Shows patience. _____	( )	( )	( )
vii. Notices cues indicating patient's discomfort and attempts to alleviate it.	( )	( )	( )
viii. Paces the procedure appropriately to tolerance and/or condition of patient. _____	( )	( )	( )
ix. Focuses attention on the procedure to the extent that readiness to respond to other events is limited. _____	( )	( )	( )
x. Indicates awareness of responsibility to the patient following procedure.	( )	( )	( )

[1] *N/A* = not applicable _____

ASSESSMENT INSTRUMENT 16

I. Check-list and rating scale: Cardiovascular examination (physician)

II. Competences to be assessed:
Data-gathering
Recording
Interpreting

III. Specific abilities to be assessed:
1. Ability to perform 76 actions involved in a cardiovascular examination.
2. Ability to interpret the data gathered during the examination.
3. Ability to conduct the examination in a thorough and professional manner.

IV. Purpose of assessment: summative.
To assess ability of medical student to carry out a cardiovascular examination and correctly interpret the signs and sounds that are observed.

V. Comments:
No evaluation has been done and no statistics are available regarding validity. Evaluator is asked to check performance for completeness and to rate the student's overall interpersonal skills.

VI. Source to contact for further information:
Dr Paula L. Stillman and Dr P. J. Rutala
Office of the Curriculum Coordinator
Preparation for Clinical Medicine
The University of Arizona
Health Sciences Center
Tucson, AZ 85724
USA

CARDIOVASCULAR EXAMINATION PERFORMANCE CHECK-LIST

Examiner's name _____

Patient's name _____

Date _____

A. *General inspection/vital signs*

_____ 1. Wash hands before starting examination.

_____ 2. Measure blood pressure in right upper limb, sitting or lying.

_____ 3. Measure blood pressure in left upper limb, sitting or lying.

_____ 4. Measure blood pressure in either upper limb, standing.

_____ 5. Empty cuff completely before inflating it.

_____ 6. Measure respiratory rate for at least 60 seconds.

_____ 7. Palpate radial pulse for at least 15 seconds.

_____ 8. Palpate radial pulse simultaneously for symmetry.

B. *Hands and arms*

_____ 1. Inspect both hands.

C. *Head and neck*

_____ 1. Palpate carotids bilaterally.

_____ 2. Auscultate carotids bilaterally.

D. *Lungs*

_____ 1. Ask patient to cross arms to move scapulae and expose lung fields.

_____ 2. Percuss posterior lung fields.

_____ 3. Percuss fields bilaterally and symmetrically, in all areas.

_____ 4. Instruct patient to breathe through open mouth.

_____ 5. Auscultate posterior lung fields.

_____ 6. Auscultate all areas bilaterally and symmetrically with patient breathing through open mouth.

Lateral lung fields

_____ 7. Percuss lateral lung fields.

_____ 8. Auscultate lateral lung fields.

Anterior lung fields

_____ 9. Percuss anterior lung fields.

_____10. Percuss fields bilaterally and symmetrically.

_____11. Auscultate anterior lung fields.

_____12. Auscultate anterior lung fields bilaterally and symmetrically.

E. *Heart*

_____ 1. Observe precordium.

Palpate with patient *sitting*:

_____ 2. Aortic area (2nd ICS-right)

_____ 3. Pulmonic area (2nd and 3rd ICS-left).

_____ 4. Right ventricular area.

_____ 5. Apical area (5th ICS left).

Auscultate with patient *sitting* (using diaphragm of stethoscope):

_____ 6. Aortic area

_____ 7. Pulmonic area

_____ 8. Tricuspid area (4th and 5th ICS at left sternal edge)

_____ 9. Mitral (apical) area.

Auscultate with patient *sitting* (using *bell* of stethoscope):

_____10. Aortic area

_____11. Pulmonic area

_____12. Tricuspid area

_____13. Apical area.

_____14. *Observe* neck veins with patient in *recumbent* position.

Palpate with patient *recumbent*:

_____15. Aortic area (2nd ICS-right)

_____16. Pulmonic area (2nd and 3rd ICS-left)

_____17. Right ventricular area.

_____18. Apical area (5th ICS-left)

_____19. Ectopic area (between right ventricular and apical areas)

Auscultate with patient *recumbent* (using diaphragm of stethoscope):

_____20. Aortic area

_____21. Pulmonic area

_____22. Tricuspid area

_____23. Mitral (apical) area.

Auscultate with patient *recumbent* (using *bell* of stethoscope):

_____24. Aortic area

_____25. Pulmonic area

_____26. Tricuspid area

_____27. Mitral (apical) area

_____28. Ask patient to roll to left lateral position.

Heart (contd.)

_____29. Relocate apex.
_____30. Auscultate apex with bell.
_____31. Auscultate apex with diaphragm.

F. Abdomen
_____ 1. Patient is taught to relax abdominal musculature.
_____ 2. Watch patient's face as you examine abdomen.
_____ 3. Auscultate before manipulation or palpation.
Auscultate
_____ 4. Aorta
_____ 5. Renal arteries
_____ 6. Iliac arteries.
_____ 7. Palpate epigastrium superficially.
_____ 8. Palpate epigastrium deeply.
_____ 9. Palpate right upper quadrant.
_____10. Use proper technique to palpate liver edge.
_____11. Percuss liver span.
_____12. Palpate left upper quadrant.
_____13. Use proper technique to palpate tip of spleen.

G. Lower limbs
_____ 1. Inspect bilaterally with outer clothes removed.
_____ 2. Inspect feet including toes.
Palpate pulses bilaterally:
_____ 3. Femoral
_____ 4. Popliteal
_____ 5. Posterior tibial
_____ 6. Dorsalis pedis.
_____ 7. Auscultate for femoral bruits.
_____ 8. Check for peripheral pitting edema.
_____ 9. Use proper technique to check for pitting edema.

Total score obtained
Total score possible 76

For the evaluator   *Key:* 5 = Always
                                    4 = Most of the time
                                    3 = Half of the time
                                    2 = Rarely
                                    1 = Never

	5	4	3	2	1
1. Did the student show concern for the patient's comfort and ensure privacy during the examination?	5	4	3	2	1
2. Did the student present himself/herself in a professional manner?	5	4	3	2	1
3. Did the student explain procedures and prepare the patient for what was being done?	5	4	3	2	1
4. Did the student perform the examination in a logical sequence, progressing from one region to another without repetition?	5	4	3	2	1
5. Did the student examine and compare symmetrical parts of the body?	5	4	3	2	1
6. Did the student use jargon not understood by the patient?	5	4	3	2	1
7. Was the examination too rough?	5	4	3	2	1

Examiner's name _____

Patient's name _____

Date _____

CARDIOVASCULAR EXAMINATION CONTENT CHECK-LIST

By having performed the 76 maneuvers of the cardiovascular examination check-list, you will now be able to answer the following questions:

Vital signs inspection
1. Blood pressure:
   (a) Right arm (sitting or lying): _____ / _____
   (b) Left arm (sitting or lying): _____ / _____
   (c) Either arm (standing): _____ / _____

2. Respiratory rate: _____ /min.

3. Radial pulse:
   (a) Rate: _____ /min.
   (b) Rhythm: regular _____ ; irregular _____
   (c) Symmetrical in both forearms? yes _____ no _____ .
       If *asymmetrical in timing*: is right pulse delayed? yes _____ no _____
                                    is left pulse delayed? yes _____ no _____
                                    estimate length of delay: _____ sec.
       If *asymmetrical in strength*, estimate (on a scale of 0–4 +):

	Right					Left		
0	1	2	3	4	0	1	2	3	4

4. Fingernail beds:
   (a) evidence of cyanosis: present _____ absent _____ .
   (b) evidence of clubbing: present _____ absent _____ .

Carotid Pulse
5. (a) Carotid pulse upstroke: normal _____ abnormal _____ .
       If abnormal: rapid _____ slow _____ .
   (b) Carotid pulse contour: normal _____ bisferiens _____ .

6. Strength of carotid pulse (estimate on a scale of 0–4 +):

	Right					Left		
0	1	2	3	4	0	1	2	3	4

7. Carotid bruits: present _____ absent _____ .
   If *present*, were bruits heard. (a) on right side? _____
                                    (b) on left side? _____ .
   If *present*, grade bruit (on a scale of 0–4 +):

	Right					Left		
0	1	2	3	4	0	1	2	3	4

Thorax and lungs
8. Pattern of percussion: normal _____ abnormal _____ .
   If *abnormal*, is it dull? _____ or hyperresonant? _____ .
   On the accompanying diagram, shade all areas of dullness and/or hyperresonance:

Posterior   Right lateral   Left lateral   Anterior

9. Rales (crackles): present _____ absent _____ .
   If *present*, the quality can be described as: fine _____ coarse _____ .
   On the accompanying diagram, shade all areas in which rales are heard:

Posterior   Right lateral   Left lateral   Anterior

10. Wheezes with quiet breathing:
    (a) present on inspiration? yes_____ no_____.
    (b) present on expiration? yes_____ no_____.
    If *present*, shade all areas on the accompanying diagram, in which wheezes are heard:

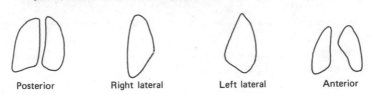

   Posterior   Right lateral   Left lateral   Anterior

Heart

11. Visible precordial motions: present_____ absent_____.
    If *present;* locate with a dark dot on the accompanying diagram:

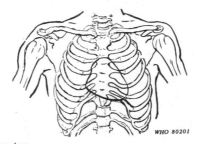

WHO 80201

12. Palpable precordial impulses:
    (a) Aortic area (2nd RICS): normal _____ hyperactive _____ sustained.
    (b) Pulmonic area (2nd LICS): normal _____ hyperactive _____ sustained _____.
    (c) Tricuspid area (4th LICS): normal _____ hyperactive _____ sustained _____.
    (d) Apical area: normal _____ hyperactive _____ sustained _____.
    (e) Palpable S4 at the apex: present _____ absent _____.
    (f) Ectopic area of precordial impulse: present _____ absent _____.
    (g) Left ventricular heave: present _____ absent _____.

13. Auscultation:
    (a) S1: single _____ _____ split _____.
    (b) Intensity of S1: normal _____ loud _____ soft _____.
    (c) S2: single _____ split _____.
       If *split*, is splitting: physiological? _____ paradoxical? _____ wide? _____ fixed? _____
    (d) Intensity of S2: normal _____ loud _____ soft _____
    (e) Intensity of pulmonic component of S2: normal _____ loud _____ soft _____.
    (f) Ejection sound heard in 2nd LICS (pulmonic area)? yes _____ no _____.
    (g) S3 present at the apex? yes _____ no _____.
    (h) S4 present at the apex? yes _____ no _____.
    (i) Midsystolic clicks: present _____ absent _____.
       if *present*: single _____ multiple _____.

14. (a) Systolic murmur(s): present _____ absent _____.
       If *present*, indicate on the accompanying diagram with a dark dot where they are *best* heard and

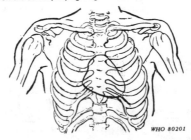

WHO 80201

(b) Grade the murmur(s) on a 1-6 + scale. Grade _____ .
(c) Do(es) murmur(s) vary with inspiration? yes _____ no _____ .
   If *yes*, do they increase? _____ or decrease? _____ .

15. (a) Diastolic murmur(s): present _____ absent _____ .
    If *present*, indicate on the accompanying diagram with a dark dot where murmur(s) are *best* heard and

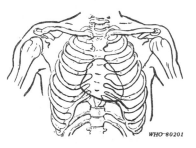

WHO 80201

(b) Grade the murmur(s) on a 1-6 + scale. Grade _____ .
(c) Do(es) murmur(s) vary with inspiration? yes _____ no _____ .
   If *yes*, do they increase? _____ or decrease? _____ .

16. Diagram all sounds heard during the cardiac cycle.

L_____|_____|_____|_____|_____|_____J

S1   S2   S1   S2   S1   S2   S1

17. Venous pressure (observed in neck veins): normal _____ ; abnormal _____ .
    If *abnormal*, is venous pulse pressure decreased? _____ or elevated? _____ .
    If *elevated*, estimate height in cm: _____ cm.

18. Abdmonial bruits heard? yes _____ no _____ .
    If *yes*, grade on a scale of 1-4 + in each area where they occur.

	Right				Left			
(a) Aorta	1	2	3	4	1	2	3	4
(b) Renal arteries	1	2	3	4	1	2	3	4
(c) Iliac arteries	1	2	3	4	1	2	3	4

19. Aorta: palpable _____ not palpable _____ .
    If *palpable*, estimate diameter in cm: _____ cm.

20. (a Overall span of liver to percussion: _____ cm.
    (b) Liver edge: palpable _____ not palpable _____ .
       If *palpable*:
       How far below the right costal margin (RCM)? _____ cm.
       tender _____ non-tender _____ .
       pulsatile _____ non-pulsatile _____ .

21. Spleen: palpable _____ not palpable _____ .
    If *palpable*, how far below the left costal margin (LCM)? _____ cm.

22. Toe nail beds:
    (a) evidence of cyanosis: present _____ absent _____ .
    (b) evidence of clubbing: present _____ absent _____ .

23. Femoral pulse:
    (a) Symmetrical strength in both groins? yes _____ no _____ .
       Grade pulse from 0 to 4 + in each groin:

	Right					Left			
0	1	2	3	4	0	1	2	3	4

24. Femoral bruits: present _____ absent _____ .
    If *present*, bruits are heard on: (a) right? yes _____ no _____ .
                                      (b) left? yes _____ no _____ .

25. Grade peripheral pulse strengths (0–4 +) for the following:

		Right					Left			
(a) popliteal pulse	0	1	2	3	4	0	1	2	3	4
(b) posterior tibial pulse	0	1	2	3	4	0	1	2	3	4
(c) dorsalis pedis pulse	0	1	2	3	4	0	1	2	3	4

26. Peripheral edema: present _____ absent _____ .
    If *present*, grade (0–4 +):

	Right limb					Left limb			
0	1	2	3	4	0	1	2	3	4

   If *present*, how far up the limb does it go (i.e., ankle, pretibial area)?
   right limb _____
   left limb _____

27. Please list any additional findings not specifically listed on this form that you feel are pertinent to the patient's condition:

28. Briefly explain the patient's underlying disease process on the basis of the abnormalities found in physical examination.

ASSESSMENT INSTRUMENT 17

I. Rating scale: Physical therapy (physical therapy assistant)

II. Competences to be assessed:
Rehabilitation training
Application of special treatments
Communication

III. Specific abilities to be assessed:
1. Ability to carry out prescribed treatment in sympathetic, professional manner.
2. Ability to prepare patient properly and adapt treatment to patient's needs.
3. Ability to prepare logical, clearly developed reports of activities.

IV. Purpose of assessment: summative.
Designed for use as final examination at end of course. Observation of practical work involved.

V. Comments:
Informal evaluation has been carried out by use and comparison with results obtained with other instruments. No statistical data available.

VI. Source to contact for further information:
Stanley Mendelson, Coordinator
Physical Therapist Assistant Program
Essex County College
375 Osborne Terrace
Newark, NJ 07112
USA

STUDENT EVALUATION FORM
(PHYSICAL THERAPY ASSISTANT)

Student's name _____

Name of supervisor _____

Name of facility _____

_____Fall   _____Winter _____Spring _____Summer _____Year

Each major objective is to be graded A, B, C, F. Several tasks are required to meet each objective: for an "A" the student must fulfill 90% of the tasks; for a "B", 80%; for a "C", 70%. Failure to achieve 70% will be graded "F".

Professional practices

1. The student conducts himself in a professional manner.   ____
   (a) Grooms himself properly, wears clean uniform and shoes.   ____
   (b) Practises personal hygiene.   ____
   (c) Shows initiative in assuming responsibility.   ____
   (d) Accepts responsibility.   ____
   (e) Assists and cooperates willingly with co-workers.   ____
   (f) Follows chain of command.   ____
   (g) Abides by regulations of facility.   ____
   (h) Uses free clinic time to advantage.   ____
   (i) Is punctual and gives advance notice of absences.   ____
   (j) Cleans treatment area after use.   ____
2. The student maintains appropriate interpersonal relationships.   ____
   (a) Reacts appropriately to the feelings of others.   ____
   (b) Shows appropriate emotional reactions in the presence of others.   ____
   (c) Contributes to a friendly but professional atmosphere.   ____
   (d) Responds favorably to criticism and suggestions.   ____
   (e) Respects confidential material.   ____
3. The student prepares for treatment.   ____
   (a) Reviews patient's medical chart.   ____
   (b) Reviews techniques of selected physical agents as necessary.   ____
   (c) Prepares area prior to treatment.   ____
   (d) Checks equipment prior to use.   ____
   (e) Drapes patient properly.   ____
4. The student applies treatment, using proper approach to patient.   ____
   (a) Instructs patient as to method and purpose of treatment.   ____
   (b) Instructs patient in proper use of physical aids.   ____
   (c) Adapts procedure to patient's needs.   ____
   (d) Practises principles of body mechanics.   ____
   (e) Notes any adverse reactions in the patient.   ____
   (f) Reports any changes in response.   ____
   (g) Treats patient within limits of tolerance (fatigue/pain).   ____
   (h) Uses and adjusts equipment properly.   ____
   (i) Follows treatment program as outlined by physical therapist.   ____
   (j) Treats patient with adequate attention to safety.   ____
5. The student prepares appropriate reports.   ____
   (a) Records results of treatments.   ____
   (b) Submits reports when indicated.   ____
   (c) Expresses ideas logically and understandably.   ____
   (d) Adapts communication to the comprehension of each individual.   ____
   (e) Uses and understands appropriate medical terminology.   ____

Please grade the following on the basis of 0–10, 7 being the minimum passing grade.

6. The student demonstrates appropriate knowledge in the following areas: ____
   (a) anatomy   ____
   (b) principles of special treatments   ____
   (c) indications   ____
   (d) contraindications   ____
   (e) dosage   ____

Please rate according to student's performance, using the following criteria:

4 Student demonstrates skill when fulfilling objective or performing technique with only guidance.

3 Student demonstrates skill when fulfilling objective or performing technique, but requires occasional supervision.

2 Student requires supervision and occasional assistance when fulfilling objective or performing technique.

1 Student is unable to fulfill objective or perform technique.

N/A Not applicable

Application of special treatments

_____ massage
_____ infrared
_____ diathermy
_____ microtherm
_____ ultrasound
_____ ultraviolet
_____ electrical stimulation
_____ cervical traction
_____ hot packs
_____ whirlpool
_____ paraffin
_____ hubbard tank

Performance of functional activities

_____ bed activities
_____ wheelchair management
_____ wheelchair transfers
_____ use of physical aids
_____ hand activities

Performance of therapeutic exercises

_____ passive and/or stretching
_____ active, active assistive
_____ progressive resistive
_____ coordination
_____ posture training
_____ neuromuscular facilitation techniques
_____ pulmonary exercises
_____ stump care
_____ stump bandaging
_____ preprosthetic training

Performance of ambulation training

_____ pre-crutch exercises
_____ stand/sit activities
_____ elevations
_____ gait training
_____ crutch measurement

Please feel free to make any comment concerning the student, the student's progress, or the program.

_____

_____

_____

_____

_____

_____

_____

Date

Supervisor's Signature

Student's Signature

ASSESSMENT INSTRUMENT 18

I. Rating scale: Anaesthetic procedures (nurse anaesthetist)

II. Competences to be assessed:
Planning and administering anaesthesia

III. Specific abilities to be assessed:
1. Ability to select anaesthetic care plan appropriate to patient's needs.
2. Ability to assemble and maintain routine and specialized anaesthetic equipment.
3. Ability to monitor vital signs and recognize mechanical or physiological problems.
4. Ability to demonstrate dexterity in carrying out anaesthesia procedures.

IV. Purpose of assessment: formative.
Used daily to assess progress of student nurse anaesthetists.

V. Comments:
In current use, and being evaluated formally by a validity workshop. No statistical data available as yet.

VI. Source to contact for further information:
Prudentia Worth, CRNA
College of Pharmacy and Allied Health Professions
Department of Anesthesia
406 Detroit General Hospital
Detroit, MI
USA

PERFORMANCE OF ANESTHETIC PROCEDURES

Student's name _____

GUIDELINES FOR RATING

Outstanding (4 points):	Exceeds required objectives, performs steps carefully and skillfully in minimal time. Is able to evaluate performance and identify ways for improvement.
Above average (3 points):	Exceeds required objectives, performs steps carefully and skillfully. Is able to evaluate performance and identify *most* of the ways for improvement. *Makes minor errors.*
Average (2 points):	Meets required objectives, demonstrates the minimally acceptable performance. Is able to identify *some* ways for improvement. *Makes major errors.*
Unsatisfactory (1 point):	Fails to meet most of the required objectives. *Makes critical errors.*

1. Statements are same for all five scales.
2. All scales have equal weight.
3. Final grades are determined from students' rating performances in all hospitals and from general observations which cannot be written into specific objectives.

Development of an anesthetic care plan	Points	Evaluation comments
1. Provides patient with a simple and reassuring explanation of visit during the pre-anesthetic assessment.		
2. Selects anesthetic care plan to meet the patient's physical and psychological needs as well as surgical requirements.		
3. Evaluates laboratory data and correctness of consent prior to developing an appropriate management plan.		
4. Analyses specific drug therapy and correlates the ASA[1] status with the pathophysiology when structuring an anesthetic plan.		
5. Determines the need for selected equipment to accommodate surgical requirement.		
6. Anticipates the need to make adjustments in the application and securing of monitoring equipment used.		
7. Chooses a cannula of appropriate size for venipuncture insertion and determines volume replacement for the individual patients and procedures.		
8. Plans induction and management based on the patient's needs, and on the type and length of the surgical procedure.		
Total		

Correlation of didactic with clinical aspects	Points	Evaluation comments
1. Correlates knowledge of pathophysiology and comprehension of anesthetic risk when assigning ASA[1] status and in making premedication recommendations.		
2. Integrates knowledge of various inhalation and intravenous anesthetics used. Determines a suitable technique for the selected case.		
3. Compares and contrasts the pharmacological effects of all relaxants used and gives reasons for specific selection.		
4. Explains mechanisms of physiological effects following positional changes and correlates knowledge to protect patient effectively.		
5. Determines the specific type of induction indicated for a given case, i.e., awake, slow, rapid, crash.		
6. Demonstrates an understanding of the principles of fluid balance and blood replacement in the patient.		
7. Distinguishes between routine oral and nasal intubation and alters technique for specific airway management problems, i.e., oral versus nasal, tube size, etc.		
8. Gives examples where preoxygenation is of critical importance in anesthetic management.		
Cumulative total		

[1] American Society of Anesthesiologists.

Implementation of anesthetic process	Points	Evaluation comments
1. Assembles and checks routine and specialized equipment. 2. Uses aseptic techniques to prepare and administer all intravenous drugs. 3. Individualizes anesthetic requirement and proceeds with appropriate induction and maintenance. 4. Assesses the need for additional laboratory data and obtains them prior to induction. 5. Demonstrates ability to chart with completeness and accuracy. 6. Uses judgement in applying and securing monitors, intravenous equipment, and face mask. 7. Positions patients, using physiological principles, and anticipates problems related to postural changes. 8. Inserts oral and nasal pharyngeal airway skillfully and demonstrates ability to recognize and correct airway problems. 9. Maintains an uncomplicated airway, coordinates ventilation, and monitors vital signs during anesthetic management. 10. Demonstrates dexterity in performing oral and nasal intubation and extubation. 11. Uses appropriate measures to assess adequate ventilation prior to extubation. 12. Administers estimated fluid requirement and assesses need for blood replacement. 13. Demonstrates ability to perform a *rapid induction* correctly. 14. Inserts esophageal stethoscope, nasogastric tube, and temperature probe skillfully and is conscious of possible complications. 15. Recognizes and attempts to make appropriate corrections of mechanical and physiological problems. 16. Identifies ECG abnormalities; attempts to determine cause and basic anesthetic adjustments. 17. Monitors vital signs, assesses the need for postoperative ventilatory support, and relays pertinent information to appropriate postanesthetic recovery staff.		
Cumulative total		

Interpersonal behavior	Points	Evaluation comments
1. Demonstrates flexibility regarding change in room or patient assignment. 2. Continuously evaluates self and recognizes capabilities and limitations. 3. Cooperative and willing to help fellow students when needed. 4. Assists with management of patients in postanesthetic recovery (arterial blood gases, extubation, monitoring, ventilatory care). 5. Demonstrates initiative in formulating anesthetic process with underclassmen. 6. Maintains effective interaction with patients, peers, and all instructional staff, including affiliated staff. 7. Shows a positive and receptive interest in all learning activities provided. 8. Demonstrates ability to respond appropriately to stressful situations.		
Cumulative total		

Care of anesthetic equipment	Points	Evaluation comments
1. Cleans and restocks all routine and specialized equipment used. 2. Turns off routine and specialized equipment, including gas supply, at end of each case. 3. Restocks drug and supply carts in emergency rooms, including the cardiac arrest cart. 4. Removes all unnecessary equipment from room after each case and reports faulty equipment. 5. Assists in the care of equipment at the end of the week.		
Cumulative total		

ASSESSMENT INSTRUMENT 19

I. Rating scale: Surgical nursing proficiency

II. Competences to be assessed:
Data-gathering
Communication
Patient-management planning
Reporting

III. Specific abilities to be assessed:
1. Ability to meet basic and special nursing needs of adult patients.
2. Ability to communicate successfully with patients and health team members.
3. Ability to infer implications for nursing from current research and events.
4. Ability to develop rapport with patients.

IV. Purpose of assessment: formative.
Used to assess clinical competence for each of two one-week modules, but highly relied on for assigning a clinical guide in the last part of the course in adult medical-surgical nursing.

V. Comments:
No evaluation data are available.

VI. Source to contact for further information:
Mary Lee S. Kirkland
Medical University of South Carolina
College of Nursing
171 Ashley Avenue
Charleston, SC 29403
USA

CLINICAL EVALUATION TOOL

Key

4 = A	Excellent	Consistently outstanding achievement	N/A = Not applicable
3 = B	Very good	Consistently above minimum expectations	N/O = Not observed
2 = C	Average	Consistently meets minimum expectations	
1 = D	Poor	Minimum expectations not met consistently	
0 = F	Fail	Unsatisfactory, unsafe performance	

Course behavior I   *Comments*

Employs the nursing process in meeting the basic and unique needs of adult clients.

Criteria: 0 1 2 3 4 N/A N/O

1. Obtains basic data on the client.

2. Identifies health problems and potential health problems.

3. Validates client problems in the clinical area.

4. Formulates goals/objectives related to identified health problems or potential health problems.

5. Formulates a plan of care for assigned clients.

6. Implements the plan of nursing care for assigned clients.

7. Evaluates the plan of nursing care daily for assigned clients.

Total points (criteria 1–7) = (   ) 4 + (   ) 3 + (   ) 2 + (   ) 1 + (   ) 0 = _____

Course behavior II

Employs communication skills in the collaborative process with members of the health team caring for adult clients.

Criteria: 0 1 2 3 4 N/A N/O

8. Discusses with other team members their goals and plans for clients so as to support or enhance those plans through nursing care.

9. Attends to clients' needs through use of referrals, both to departments within the hospital and to other community agencies.

10. Informs other team members of progress (or lack of progress) towards meeting goals/objectives for clients in order to ensure continuity.

11. Uses therapeutic interviewing techniques to obtain subjective data from clients.

Total points (criteria 8–11) = (   ) 4 + (   ) 3 + (   ) 2 + (   ) 1 + (   ) 0 = _____

Course behavior III

Utilizes selected current research findings in approaches to nursing intervention for adult clients.

Criterion: 0 1 2 3 4 N/A N/O

12. Demonstrates the use of research findings in planning and/or examining the rationale for nursing intervention.

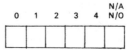

Course behavior IV

Explores current health-related events and their implications for professional growth and action in adult nursing.

Criterion:

	0	1	2	3	4	N/A N/O
13. Submits in writing a critique of a specified activity.						

Total points (criteria 12–13) = ( ) 4 +( ) 3 +( ) 2 +( ) 1 +( ) 0 = _____

Course behavior V

Combines responsibility and accountability in providing health care for adult clients.

Criteria:

	0	1	2	3	4	N/A N/O
14. Supports routines and regulations of health care system and facilitates compromise when goals of the client and health care system are in conflict.						
15. Reports to the clinical unit prepared to care for assigned client(s).						
16. Records all pertinent information concisely and legibly on chart, Kardex, and medical records.						
17. Verbally reports significant observations to charge nurse or nursing staff member caring for client.						

Total points (criteria 14–17) = ( ) 4 +( ) 3 +( ) 2 +( ) 1 +( ) 0 = _____

Course behavior VI

Incorporates knowledge of self and self-direction in interpersonal relationships and learning situations.

Criteria:

	0	1	2	3	4	N/A N/O
18. Recognizes individual learning needs and avails self of opportunities for learning.						
19. Is self-directing in providing care to clients.						
20. Creates an atmosphere of mutual trust, acceptance, and respect.						

Total points (criteria 18–20) = ( ) 4 +( ) 3 +( ) 2 +( ) 1 +( ) 0 = _____

Course behavior VII

Applies knowledge of principles and theories from the sciences and humanities in nursing care of the adult client.

Criteria:

	0	1	2	3	4	N/A N/O
21. Discusses in clinical conference theoretical knowledge related to the client's problems.						
22. Utilizes knowledge of medication in administering care to clients.						
23. Integrates into nursing care knowledge of major health problems and stressors affecting the adult population.						
24. Utilizes knowledge of the teaching-learning process in the care of clients.						
25. Integrates knowledge of causation and prevention and treatment procedures in the care of clients with injuries or illnesses requiring immediate attention.						

Total points (criteria 21–25) = ( ) 4 +( ) 3 +( ) 2 +( ) 1 +( ) 0 = _____

Cumulative points_____   Average_____

ASSESSMENT INSTRUMENT 20

I. Check-list: Physical examination—heart, lungs, abdomen (physician's assistant)

II. Competences to be assessed:
Data-gathering
Physical assessment

III. Specific types of ability to be assessed:
1. Ability to differentiate normal from abnormal structure and function.
2. Ability to detect and identify signs and sounds of physical abnormalities.

IV. Purpose of assessment: formative.
Used periodically during course for physician's assistant training. Designed to evaluate physical examination performance.

V. Comments:
No formal evaluation has been performed and no data are available on validity.

VI. Source to contact for further information:
Stephen C. Gladhart
Program Director
Physician Assistant Program
Wichita State University
VA Center Building 5
5500 E. Kellogg
Wichita, KS
USA

PHYSICAL EXAMINATION OF THE HEART

Yes   No

1. Instructed the patient about procedure.
2. Exposed chest to reveal landmarks.
3. Placed the patient in sitting position and performed the following:
4. *Inspection*
   (*a*) Any abnormal pulsations?
   (*b*) Is point of maximum intensity visible, localized, or diffuse, location by interspace and distance from left sternal border or mid-clavicular line?
5. *Palpation*
   (*a*) Placed hand over 2nd interspace to right of the sternum.
   (*b*) Placed hand over 2nd interspace to the left of sternum.
   (*c*) Placed hand over the apical area.
   (*d*) Palpated the apex beat, noted intensity, measured the location of the apex beat by interspace and distance from the left border of the sternum or from mid-clavicular line.
6. *Auscultation*
   (*a*) Were heart rate and regularity determined over the apex and checked with radial pulse?
   (*b*) Was auscultation with bell and diaphragm performed in the following areas?
   (1) The apical area, left lateral position.
   (2) 2nd right interspace and Erb's point.
   (3) 2nd left interspace.
   (4) Area just above the xiphoid.
   (5) When Erb's point was auscultated, was patient requested to lean forward and exhale deeply?
   (*c*) Ask student to describe abnormalities.
   (*d*) Was abnormality validated by supervising examiner?

EXAMINATION OF THE LUNGS

Yes   No

1. Instructed patient about procedure.
2. Exposed the chest to reveal landmarks.
3. Placed the patient in a sitting position and performed the following.
4. *Inspection*
   (*a*) Counted respiratory rate per minute.
   (*b*) Noted amplitude of breathing: shallow, deep, normal.
   (*c*) Noted respiratory rhythm: regular, irregular, periodic.
   (*d*) Noted chest deformities, symmetry, the use of accessory muscles of respiration
   (*e*) Noted degree of chest expansion using measuring tape.
5. *Palpation*
   (*a*) Noted degree of chest expansion bilaterally by placing hands on lower thoracic cage, both anterior and posterior, having patient inhale and exhale deeply.
   (*b*) Elicited tactile fremitus.
6. *Percussion*
   (*a*) Anterior lung fields, upper, bilaterally.
   (*b*) Lateral lung fields.
   (*c*) Posterior lung fields, upper, middle, and lower.
7. *Auscultation*
   (*a*) Anterior upper lung fields for vocal fremitus.
   (*b*) Lateral lung fields, asking patient to breathe more deeply and rapidly with mouth open.
   (*c*) Posterior lung fields, upper, mid, and lower, asking the patient to breathe more deeply and rapidly with mouth open.
   (*d*) Is each area auscultated for intensity and duration of inspiration and expiration and the presence or absence of adventitious sounds, with the patient inhaling and exhaling deeply through his mouth?
   (*e*) Is the patient requested to cough after a deep expiration as a part of auscultation?
   (*f*) Are pectoriloquy and vocal fremitus performed?

PHYSICAL EXAMINATION OF THE ABDOMEN

Yes   No

1. Instructed the patient about procedure.
2. Exposed the abdomen to the extent that the four quadrants were revealed.
3. Placed patient in supine position.
4. Placed patient's arms to his side or on his chest.
5. *Inspection*
   (a) Was abdomen carefully inspected for type, presence of distention, dermatitis, abnormal pulsations or masses, scars, venous engorgement, protusion in flanks?
6. *Auscultation*
   (a) Was auscultation performed over the four quadrants of the abdomen and the renal areas posterior?
7. *Percussion*
   (a) Was percussion performed over the four quadrants of the abdomen and any abnormality described by location, size, shape?
   (b) Demonstrated the tests for shifting dullness in the supine position.
   (c) Demonstrated the tests for shifting dullness in the lateral position.
   (d) Have student demonstrate how the succussion splash is elicited.
8. *Palpation*
   (a) Was patient requested to report tenderness or pain when palpating?
   (b) Was palpation performed in the four quadrants initially superficially and then deeply for tenderness, pain, rigidity, guarding, masses, hernia, and adequately described? Location, size, and shape, consistency, texture (smooth or modular), movable or nonmovable, pulsatile.
9. *Liver*
   (a) Percussed upper liver border.
   (b) Palpated by placing left hand under the patient.
   (c) Asked patient to take deep breath while palpating lower edge by moving from right lower quadrant to right upper quadrant.
   (d) Was lower edge of liver palpated in the medial line?
   (e) If liver edge palpable, measured span between upper and lower borders and from lower costal margin to liver edge.
10. *Spleen*
    (a) When palpating placed one hand under patient. Asked patient to take deep breath while palpating, moving from left lower quadrant to left upper quadrant.
    (b) Patient rolled to the right at approximately 30 degrees and lower edge of spleen palpated.
    (c) Lower edge of spleen palpated with thighs flexed at approximately 45 degrees.
11. *Kidneys*
    (a) Lower edge of kidneys palpated bilaterally.
13. Did the student find any abnormalities?
14. Was the student standing on right side of patient?
15. Were these abnormalities verified by the supervising examiner?

ASSESSMENT INSTRUMENT 21

I. Rating scale: Specific nursing activities

II. Competences to be assessed:
Clinical skills
— hanging and monitoring an intravenous drip (IV)
— administering "piggyback" medications
— change of dressing
— application of elastic bandages
— protective isolation
— isolation
— urinary bladder catheterization
— tracheal suctioning
Communication

III. Specific abilities to be assessed:
1. Abilities required to perform the nursing care techniques listed above.

IV. Purpose of assessment: summative.
Used periodically as each technique is learned, and/or as final examination at end of nursing course.

V. Comments:
Instrument has not been evaluated. Each part affords step by step analysis of the relevant technique.

VI. Source to contact for further information:
Colleen A. Martin
Director
School of Nursing
Grand Valley State College
Allendale, MI. 49417
USA

EVALUATION FORMS FOR SPECIFIC TECHNIQUES
Hanging and monitoring an intravenous drip (IV)

The student will perform the following steps in preparing and hanging an IV.

Behavior	Points possible	Points earned
1. Chooses correct solution from stock supply as determined directly from physician's order.	10	
2. Calculates correct drip rate to implement physician's order.	15	
3. Checks bottle/solution for cracks, impurities, and expiration date.	10	
4. Labels bottle with:		
(a) client's name		
(b) date and time started	5	
(c) sequence of bottle	5	
(d) student's name and initials	5	
(e) number of cc/h	5	
(f) number of gtt/min.	5	
5. Identifies client by comparing ID band with bottle label.	10	
6. Hangs new bottle by connecting into existing tubing set-up, maintaining surgical asepsis.	15	
7. Using the regulator clamp below the drip chamber, adjusts drip rate to within 3 gtt/min. of calculated rate.	10	
TOTAL	100	

COMMENTS:

Instructor's signature _____ Date_____

Student's signature _____ Date_____

Administering "piggyback" medications

The student will perform the following steps in demonstrating administration of "piggyback" medications.
Read pertinent information on drug before final examination.
Physician's order:

Behavior	Points possible	Points earned
1. Chooses correct medicament as determined by physician's order.	10	
2. Determines safe rate for infusion of medicament on basis of literature.	10	
3. Checks bag for impurities, leaks, and expiration date.	10	
4. Identifies client by comparing ID band with label.	10	
5. Checks infusion site for redness, swelling, tenderness, and patency.	10	
6. Hangs new bag, clears tubing and needle of air.	10	
7. Hangs medication bag higher than main bag, using metal hanger.	5	
8. Cleanses rubber intake area of main system and inserts needle.	5	
9. Opens regulator clamp of medication bag as completely as possible.	5	
10. Regulates drip rate using main system regulator clamp with 3 gtt min.	5	
Assuming that all the medicament has been infused:		
11. Closes regulator clamp of medication bag completely.	5	
12. Re-regulates drip rate of main system to recorded rate within 3 gtt min.	5	
13. States has recorded drug, dose, solution, amount of solution, route, and time.	5	
14. States has recorded amount of solution infused	5	
TOTAL	100	

COMMENTS:

Instructor's signature _____ Date_____

Student's signature _____ Date_____

Change of dressing

The student will perform the following steps in demonstrating change of dressing.

Behavior	Points possible	Points earned
1. Preparation		
(a) Explains procedure to client.	5	
(b) Checks appearance of present dressing.	5	
(c) Washes hands.	5	
(d) Obtains necessary equipment.	5	
1. 4 × 4's		
2. abdominal (ABD) pad		
3. tape		
4. waterproof bag		
5. sterile gloves		
6. non-sterile glove		
(e) Prepares lengths of tape.	2	
(f) Arranges equipment.	3	
(g) Opens sterile packages.	5	
(h) Positions client and provides for privacy.	5	
2. Removes soiled dressings		
(a) Removes tape from old dressing, stabilizing skin.	5	
(b) Removes soiled dressings. Wears non-sterile glove or uses forceps.	5	
(c) Discards soiled dressings in waterproof bag.	5	
3. Applies sterile dressing, maintaining surgical asepsis:		
(a) Dons sterile gloves.	10	
(b) Uses 4 × 4's to dry skin around wound as necessary.	10	
(c) Fluffs 4 × 4 and applies to wound.	10	
(d) Applies ABD pad.	5	
(e) Places tape parallel to major body folds.	10	
4. Records observations (states what would be recorded)	5	
(a) degree of healing		
(b) presence and amount of inflammation and/or necrotic tissue.		
(c) color and odor of drainage.		
(d) condition of sutures and drains, if present.		
TOTAL	100	

COMMENTS:

Instructor's signature _____ Date_____

Student's signature _____ Date_____

Application of elastic bandages

The student will perform the following steps in demonstrating the application of elastic bandages to a leg.

Behavior	Points possible	Points earned
1. Prior to application, assesses circulatory status of extremity (states how nurse would do this).	10	
2. Applies bandage from distal to proximal.	10	
3. Makes one circular wrap around foot to secure bandage.	10	
4. Brings second wrap around ankle and back to foot in "figure 8" wrap.	10	
5. Third wrap is made from foot to ankle and back, covering heel.	10	
6. Continues with "figure 8" wrap to thigh.	10	
7. Maintains consistent moderate pressure while wrapping.	10	
8. Checks back of knee to avoid excessive pressure.	10	
9. Places fingers under wrap while applying clips.	5	
10. Secures bandage by placing tape strip on entire length of bandage.	5	
11. Checks circulatory status of foot after application of bandage.	10	
TOTAL	100	

COMMENTS:

Instructor's signature _____ Date_____

Student's signature _____ Date_____

Protective isolation

Behavior	Points possible	Points earned
A. Entering a protective isolation area		
1. After washing hands, turns off faucet handles with dry paper towel.	10	
2. Applies necessary garments		
(a) Applies hair-covering so all hair is secured/covered.	10	
(b) Applies mask so nose and mouth are covered.	10	
(c) Re-washes hands; turns off faucet with dry paper towel.	10	
(d) Applies gown so that "client contact" areas remain uncontaminated (partner secures ties).	10	
(e) Applies gloves, using aseptic technique.	10	
(f) Applies gloves so that the gown cuffs are covered by the glove cuffs.	10	
3. Explains method of entering room without contamination of self.	10	
B. Admitting an article to the protective isolation area (partner outside room stands at door with article partially unwrapped)		
1. Directs the transfer of an article in such a way that neither the article nor the "inside" nurse's apparel are contaminated.	10	
C. Leaving a protective isolation area		
1. On leaving, removes garments and discards in receptacle outside protective isolation room.	10	
TOTAL	100	

COMMENTS:

Instructor's signature _____ Date_____

Student's signature _____ Date_____

Isolation ("bagging-out" and leaving room)

The student will perform the following steps in demonstrating isolation technique.

Behavior	Points possible	Points earned
1. "Bagging-out"		
(a) Seals the bag of contaminated linen.	5	
(b) Places the sealed bag upside down in the clean bag (being held by a colleague).	5	
(c) Does not touch the outside of the clean bag or the colleague with contaminated gloves or gown.	10	
2. Leaving the room		
(a) With gloves on, unties the waist strings of the gown.	5	
(b) Removes and discards gloves.	5	
(c) Washes hands.	10	
(d) Unties neck strings of gown.	5	
(e) Removes gown, keeping clean side of gown toward self.	5	
(f) Grasps gown on the inside and turns contaminated surfaces together.	5	
(g) Holds gown away from uniform and folds it from neck down.	5	
(h) Does not allow contaminated surfaces of gown to come in contact with uniform. Discards gown.	10	
(i) Washes hands and forearms.	5	
(j) Turns off faucet with paper towel. Discards.	5	
(k) Removes mask by strings on elastic and deposits in trash.	5	
(l) Opens door by using clean paper towel.	5	
(m) Discards paper towel in waste receptacle *inside* unit.	10	
TOTAL	100	

COMMENTS:

Instructor's signature _____ Date_____

Student's signature _____ Date_____

Urinary bladder catheterization

The student will perform the following steps in performing a female urinary bladder catheterization.
Note: Client has already been positioned, draped, and washed. The procedure has been explained to her.

Behavior	Points possible	Points earned
1. Exposes client's perineum.	5	
2. Opens catheter set, using aseptic technique.*	10	
3. Places sterile drape under buttocks.*	10	
4. Dons sterile gloves.*	10	
5. Pours sterile solution over cotton balls.*	10	
6. Tests catheter balloon.*	5	
7. Lubricates catheter.*	10	
8. Using forceps, cleanses labia and meatus with sterile cotton balls.*	10	
9. Uses sterile glove to insert catheter into meatus, 5–7 cm.*	10	
10. Holds catheter in place while inflating balloon.	10	
11. Tests for placement of catheter.	5	
12. Properly secures catheter by taping to inner thigh.	5	
TOTAL	100	

* Maintains aseptic technique during these steps.

COMMENTS:

Instructor's signature _____ Date_____

Student's signature _____ Date_____

Tracheal suctioning

The student will perform the following steps in tracheal suctioning.

Behavior	Points possible	Points earned
'1. Washes hands.	3	
2. Gathers equipment (saline, suction package, source of suction) and checks suction setting.	2	
3. Explains procedure to client.	5	
4. Prepares suction package, opens using sterile technique.	5	
5. Puts normal saline in cup properly.	5	
6. Puts sterile glove on dominant hand.	5	
7. Attaches sterile catheter to suction.	5	
8. Lubricates catheter with normal saline.	5	
9. Tells client that placement of catheter will occur.	5	
10. Gently and quickly puts catheter down as far as can go.	5	
11. Suction is *not* applied while catheter is being inserted.	10	
12. Pulls catheter back 1–2 cm.	5	
13. Applies intermittent suction while removing catheter.	10	
14. Rotates or twirls catheter while removing catheter.	10	
15. Catheter withdrawal done in 5–10 seconds.	10	
16. States that he/she will allow client to rest before repeating procedure.	3	
17. Assesses client after suctioning (states each step of assessment).	5	
(a) general color		
(b) color of nailbeds		
(c) lung sounds		
(d) reaction of client (anxiety, combativeness, etc.).		
18. Records observations (states that would be recorded).	2	
(a) assessment data		
(b) color of secretions		
(c) type or consistency of secretions		
(d) amount of secretions		
TOTAL	100	

COMMENTS:

Instructor's signature _____ Date_____

Student's signature _____ Date_____

ASSESSMENT INSTRUMENT 22

I. Check-list: Paediatric cardiac catheterization (physician)

II. Competences to be assessed:
Patient-care planning
Catheterization skills
Communication

III. Specific types of ability to be assessed:
1. Ability to plan and carry out appropriate cardiac-catheter study.
2. Ability to prepare comprehensive report of study results.
3. Ability to select and inspect the appropriate catheter and other essential equipment.
4. Ability to manipulate equipment and manage complications as they occur.

IV. Purpose of assessment: summative.
Used as final examination for medical students in paediatric cardiology.

V. Comments:
No reported use since 1972. No evaluations have been done, hence no statistical data on validity.

VI. Source to contact for further information:
Sandra Lass
Department of Medical Education
University of Southern California School of Medicine
1975 Zonal Avenue
Los Angeles, CA 90033
USA

PEDIATRIC CARDIOLOGY CARDIAC CATHETERIZATION RATING FORM

Part I. Pre- and post-catheterization considerations

____Left heart catheter
____Right heart catheter

Pre-catheterization preparations	Equipment check and selection
____Reviews patient's history. ____Evaluates physical findings. ____States the indications for the study. ____Personally evaluates the patient to check for contraindications such as anemia, fever, infections, etc.	Inspects and checks for availability of: ____balanced manometers ____calibrated oximeters ____fluoroscopy ____equipment for measuring pH level ____equipment for measuring hemoglobin.
Prepares a plan which includes: ____type of catheterization to be performed ____site of injection ____type of information to be obtained ____method of obtaining information ____pre-catheterization orders (e.g., medication).	Checks for availability and inspects: ____electrical defibrillator ____laryngoscope ____anesthesia bag type of unit ____suctioning equipment ____oxygen ____emergency drugs. ____endotracheal tubes
Communicates with house staff: ____type of catheterization to be performed ____site of injection ____type of information to be obtained ____method of obtaining information ____pre-catheterization orders (e.g., medication).	____Selects the appropriate catheter with respect to vessel size, size of patient, and type of catheter. Comments:
____Informs the parent and patient (if appropriate) of reason for and nature of the catheter study.	

Post-catheterization review	
Provides post-catheterization orders for: ____bleeding ____pulse rate and blood pressure ____other special needs.	Name _____ Key: (+) Yes Observer's name _____ (−) No Date _____ (NA) Not applicable (I) Intervened
____Notifies the parents as to whether or not needed data were obtained.	
____Makes arrangements for conference with parents for review of data.	
Prepares a comprehensive report which includes: ____data analysis (flows, output, valve areas) ____recommendations and comments ____communication with referring physician or cardiovascular surgeon.	

PEDIATRIC CARDIOLOGY CARDIAC CATHETERIZATION RATING FORM

Part II. Catheterization performance

____ Left heart catheter
____ Right heart catheter

Catheter manipulation	Special patient considerations
____ Inspects the catheter for breaks and flexibility. ____ Test-flushes the catheter. ____ Uses adequate local anesthetic. ____ Is able to insert catheter. ____ Avoids looping or knotting of catheter. ____ Is able to manipulate catheter to locations critical to making an accurate diagnosis. ____ Comments on normal and abnormal features of chambers and vessels of heart as he moves catheter from one location to another. ____ Removes catheter satisfactorily.	Comments on changes (if any) in: ____ heart rate and rhythm ____ blood pressure ____ skin color ____ respiration ____ pH level ____ airway patency. ____ Determines blood loss prior to removal of catheter. ____ Replaces blood prior to removal of catheter (if necessary). ____ Determines other abnormal conditions (if any) that require correction prior to removal of catheter.
	Selective angiography
	____ Selects the appropriate volume of contrast material ____ Test-injects for safety Injects at the appropriate sites: ____ pressures ____ volume rate of blood flow. Obtains optimal film coverage: ____ duration of filming ____ speed of filming. ____ Interprets angiographic data adequately.
Data collection	*Management of complications*
Collects appropriate blood sample data: ____ at the appropriate locations ____ of adequate size with respect to child ____ in adequate numbers of samples. Takes appropriate pressure recordings ____ at the appropriate locations ____ at basal states ____ in adequate numbers. ____ Makes appropriate use of fluoroscopy Elicits from staff on a continuous basis: ____ pressure data ____ O_2 saturation. ____ Assesses cardiac output. ____ Plans for selective studies.	Manipulates catheter into: ____ coronary sinus ____ around papillary muscle ____ ventricular sinusoid ____ coronary artery ____ pulmonary vein ____ other (please specify): _____ ____ atrial appendage. ____ Removes catheter from potentially hazardous locations. ____ Encounters complications. Manages complications successfully (if they occur).

ASSESSMENT INSTRUMENT 23

I. Rating scale: Proficiency in respiratory therapy

II. Competences to be assessed:
Communication
Case management
Recording

III. Specific types of ability to be assessed:
1. Ability to determine patients' physiological values as a baseline for treatment.
2. Ability to initiate and modify therapy as needed.
3. Ability to record essential data on medical record.
4. Ability to communicate effectively with patient and physician.

IV. Purpose of assessment: formative.
Used periodically during training of respiratory therapists.

V. Comments:
Evaluated by specialist in tests and measurements. Validity and reliability studies in progress and will be available.

VI. Source to contact for further information:
Shelley Cominsky
Respiratory Therapy Department
School of Allied Health
Medical College of Georgia
1407 Laney-Walker Boulevard
Augusta, GA 30902
USA

RESPIRATORY THERAPY

Performance rating scale 0 = Omission of step—required task not performed 1 = Unacceptable—one or more life-threatening or therapy-compromising errors 2 = Acceptable—two or less non-life-threatening errors or errors that do *not* compromise therapy 3 = Above average—no errors *Attitude rating scale* (to be used *only* by the instructor who witnesses the student's performance) 0 = Negative—easily frustrated and uncooperative 1 = Generally negative—easily frustrated *or* uncooperative 2 = Generally positive—tolerates frustration, cooperative 3 = Positive—cheerful, congenial, tolerates frustration, very cooperative	Performance rating score	Rater's assessment of step (check one)			Student _____ Evaluator _____ Overall score _____ Attitude score _____ *Justification of score and comments*
		Very important	Important	Unimportant	
1. Examination of record 　(*a*) verify doctor's orders 　(*b*) establish diagnosis 　(*c*) indication for therapy 　(*d*) evaluate for possible contraindication 2. Collect equipment 　(*a*) per order 3. Pre-mix medication 4. Introduce yourself 5. Identify patient 7. Assemble equipment and check for proper functions 8. Place patient in proper position 9. Establish baseline physiological values 　(*a*) pulse 　(*b*) blood pressure 　(*c*) breath sounds 　(*d*) observation of WOB ("work of breathing") 　(*e*) color 10. Initiate therapy, adjusting control setting and patient breathing pattern as necessary 11. Assess response to therapy 　(*a*) vital signs 　(*b*) breath sounds 　(*c*) WOB 12. Remodify control setting and patient breathing pattern as necessary 13. Terminate treatment at appropriate time 14. Reposition patient if necessary and solicit cough 15. Instruct patient about the after-effects of treatment 16. Reposition patient 17. Reassess vital signs and breath sounds if appropriate 18. Disassemble circuit and respirator 19. Wash hands 20. Locate and record procedures, results, and patient response on patient's medical record 21. Communicate with physician if necessary					

ASSESSMENT INSTRUMENT 24

I. Check-list: Proficiency in radiation oncology technology (radiation therapist)

II. Competences to be assessed:
Case management
Radiation procedures

III. Specific types of ability to be assessed:
1. Ability to interpret instructions correctly and operate assigned equipment safely and efficiently.
2. Ability to position patients appropriately and provide for their comfort.

IV. Purpose of assessment: formative.
Used periodically during training of radiation therapy technologists. Currently in use.

V. Comments:
No evaluation has been done, nor are data available concerning validity.

VI. Source to contact for further information:
Dr Jerry Gates
School of Health Sciences
Michael Reese Hospital and Medical Center
530 East 31st Street
Chicago, IL 60616
USA

RADIATION ONCOLOGY
CLINICAL EVALUATION

Rotation I

(Weeks 1–17)

Student _____ Location_____

	Yes	No
1. Does the student handle the patients and ensure their comfort appropriately?		
2. Can the student set the field size correctly?		
3. Can the student set the gantry angle correctly?		
4. Can the student set the treatment distance correctly?		
5. Can the student set the treatment table correctly?		
6. Is the student aware of, and able to implement, all radiation safety procedures?		
7. Does the student understand the purpose and importance of skin markings?		
8. Can the student correctly operate the control panel under supervision?		
9. Is the student starting to recognize common behavioral patterns in the cancer patients?		
10. Does the student maintain cleanliness and order in the treatment room?		
11. Can the student correctly identify body planes and anatomical terms necessary for the treatment set-up?		
12. Can the student correctly interpret the set-up instructions?		
13. Can the student operate the assigned equipment under supervision?		
14. Is the student starting to perform darkroom procedures?		
15. Can the student assist in all filming techniques (localization, verification, and diagnostic)?		
16. Can the student use his knowledge of body planes, anatomical terms, etc. to prepare patients for examination?		

Supervisory comments:

Student's comments:

Evaluator's signature _____

Student's signature _____

Recommended grade for rotation_____

ASSESSMENT INSTRUMENT 25

I. Rating scale: Patient education (physician's assistant)

II. Competence to be assessed:
Communication with patients

III. Specific abilities to be assessed:
1. Ability to establish rapport with patient.
2. Ability to transmit essential information in understandable form.
3. Ability to provide effective follow-up procedures.

IV. Purpose of assessment: formative.
Used in physician's assistant programme to assess ability to teach some aspect of health behaviour to a simulated patient.

V. Comments:
Instrument is new and in process of revision. No evaluation data available as yet. First used early in 1979.

VI. Source to contact for further information:
Henry Stoll and Martha Duhamel
MEDEX Northwest
University of Washington
Seattle, WA
USA

PATIENT EDUCATION

OBSERVATION SHEET

Student's name _____

Protocol topic _____

Observer's name _____

Performance feedback Did the student:	+ +	+	−	Not observed	Comments or examples
(a) Establish rapport with patient?					
(b) Determine patient's level of interest and/or readiness for learning about topic?					
(c) Find out what patient already knows, using open-ended, focused questions?					
(d) Provide new information in manner that seemed to be understood by patient? e.g.,					
1. clarity of language (jargon?)					
2. systematic (logical) sequence of ideas and concepts					
3. use of pertinent examples, analogies, or applications					
4. appropriate depth for patient's intellectual/emotional level					
5. recognize patient's saturation point (know when to stop).					
(e) Determine whether patient understood information, using effective ("non-regurgitative") questioning?					
(f) Use visual aids appropriately?					
(g) Give patient a handout or reinforce information in some other way?					
(h) Offer a method of follow-up for problems or confusion at home (e.g., "please call me . . .")?					
PROTOCOL FEEDBACK: How well does written protocol convey content and process used?					

ASSESSMENT INSTRUMENT 26

I. Check-list: Dental hygiene procedures (dental hygienist)

II. Competences to be assessed:
Data-gathering
Recording
Patient management
Patient education
Scaling of teeth

III. Specific types of ability to be assessed:
1. Ability to elicit relevant medical-dental history.
2. Ability to carry out extra- and intra-oral examinations and record resulting data accurately.
3. Ability to instruct patient in techniques of brushing teeth and using floss.
4. Ability to scale teeth effectively and efficiently.
5. Ability to perform dental hygiene procedures in accordance with acceptable professional standards.

IV. Purpose of assessment: summative.
Used periodically to assess ability in areas of the preliminary dental examination; patient education; and scaling techniques.

V. Comments:
No evaluation has been done.

VI. Source to contact for further information:
Mary C. Ward
Department of Dental Hygiene
School of Health Related Professions
University of Mississippi Medical Center
2500 State Street
Jackson, MS 39216
USA

PERFORMANCE OF DENTAL HYGIENE PROCEDURES

Student _____   Possible total _____100_____
Instructor _____
Date _____   Total _____
Patient _____

Preliminary examination

_____ 1. Reviews with patient, the medical/dental history and makes notes of positive responses. (15)
_____ 2. Positions patient and self for maximum visibility. (5)
_____ 3. Completes extra-oral and intra-oral examination.
_____   (a) Uses systematic order of inspection. (5)
_____   (b) Records accurately, using defined abbreviations and symbols. (10)
_____   (c) Palpates lymph nodes and oral mucosa and salivary glands correctly to identify non-normal consistency, and records condition. (15)
_____   (d) Visually inspects gingiva, lips, oral mucosa, tonsillar region, and tongue and records condition. (15)
_____   (e) Examines occlusion and temporomandibular joint (TMJ) function and records condition. (5)
_____   (f) Examines oral hygiene and makes note of condition. (5)
_____ 4. Takes blood pressure measurement and pulse and makes note on record. (8)
_____ 5. Takes precautions to prevent disease transmission and prevent need for emergency care. (2)
_____ 6. Plans treatment to suit patient's needs. (5)
_____ 7. Uses clinic time wisely. (2)
_____ 8. Demonstrates consideration for patient. (2)
_____ 9. Presents an acceptable personal appearance. (2)
_____10. Maintains neat and clean surgery. (2)
_____11. Demonstrates professional attitude and conforms to the code of ethics. (2)
   Comments:

Student _____   Possible total _____100_____
Instructor _____
Date _____   Total _____
Patient _____

Patient education

_____ 1. Identifies patient's needs.
_____   (a) Developes adequate rapport. (8)
_____   (b) Discloses plaque. (5)
_____   (c) Evaluates Oral Hygiene Index. (5)
_____   (d) Demonstrates area of accumulation to patient. (5)
_____ 2. Communicates on patient's level. (15)
_____ 3. Demonstrates proper floss technique.
_____   (a) Explains purpose and need. (5)
_____   (b) Demonstrates technique. (b)
_____   (c) Has patient perform technique. (5)
_____   (d) Corrects patient's technique as necessary. (5)
_____ 4. Demonstrates proper brushing technique.
_____   (a) Describes proper brushing technique. (5)
_____   (b) Positions bristles properly, using correct angle. (5)
_____   (c) Uses correct stroke. (5)
_____   (d) Establishes sequence. (5)
_____ 5. Uses educational aids when indicated. (5)
_____ 6. Designs home care program to meet patient's needs. (5)
_____ 7. Uses clinic time wisely. (2)
_____ 8. Demonstrates consideration for patient. (2)
_____ 9. Presents an acceptable personal appearance. (2)
_____10. Maintains neat and clean surgery. (2)
_____11. Demonstrates professional attitude and conforms to the code of ethics. (2)
_____12. Uses sterile technique. (2)
   Comments:

Student _____   Possible total ____100____

Instructor _____

Date _____   Total _____

Patient _____

Quadrant or area _____

          (designated by instructor)

Scaling

_____ 1. Uses correct patient-operator position. (4)

_____ 2. Uses mouth mirror, dental light, and compressed air to obtain maximum visibility. (3)

_____ 3. Uses correct instrument. (10)

_____ 4. Adapts and angles blade to tooth surface correctly, and activates correct stroke. (10)

_____ 5. Works into interproximal area. (5)

_____ 6. Maintains control and fulcrum. (8)

_____ 7. Uses sharp instruments. (5)

_____ 8. Uses good wrist-arm movement. (5)

_____ 9. Uses systematic approach. (5)

_____10. Does not lacerate soft tissue. (8)

_____11. Effectively removes deposits. (25)

_____12. Uses clinic time wisely. (2)

_____13. Demonstrates consideration for patient. (2)

_____14. Presents an acceptable personal appearance. (2)

_____15. Maintains neat and clean surgery. (2)

_____16. Demonstrates professional attitude and conforms to the code of ethics. (2)

_____17. Uses sterile technique. (2)

          Comments:

ASSESSMENT INSTRUMENT 27

I. Check-list: Maternity care (traditional birth attendant)

II. Competences to be assessed:
Antenatal care
Delivery
Care of newborn
Postpartum care

III. Specific types of ability to be assessed:
1. Ability to recognize onset of labour and prepare for delivery properly.
2. Ability to monitor normal progress during birth and perform safe, hygienic delivery
3. Ability to provide appropriate postpartum care of mother and infant.

IV. Purpose of assessment: Summative.
Comprehensive evaluation of total tasks involved in delivery.

V. Comments:
Developed to assess the traditional birth attendant's performance of a delivery in a home setting.

VI. Source:
Traditional birth attendants. Geneva, World Health Organization, 1979 (WHO Offset Publication, No. 44), pages 70–73.

Sample checklist to assess a TBA's performance during
a delivery demonstration in the home

| Name of TBA _____ | Observed by _____ |
| Location of TBA _____ | Date of observation _____ |

	Performance			Comment
	Plus*	Minus*	N.O.*	
A. Recognition of onset of labour				
1. Inquires about the presence and duration of				
- backache or abdominal cramps				
- pink discharge or "show"				
- uterine contractions				
- breaking of "bag of waters"				
2. Examines the abdomen to determine				
- position of baby				
- duration of contractions				
- severity of contractions				
B. Preparation for delivery				
1. Selects site for the delivery that is				
- quiet, clean, ventilated				
- uncluttered,with adequate space for arranging supplies				
2. Prepares equipment for the delivery				
- scrubs hands				
- removes contents of delivery kit				
- boils scissors 10 minutes				
- arranges items for easy reachability				
- covers supplies with clean cover until ready for use during delivery				
- obtains container for waste				
- covers delivery site with clean material				
3. Prepares herself for delivery				
- covers hair				
- scrubs hands thoroughly prior to preparation of mother				
- performs additional hand-scrubbing as necessary during delivery				
- puts on clean apron or the like when delivery is near				
4. Prepares mother for delivery				
- checks if mother bathed early in labour				
- helps mother to bathe if needed				
- cleanses vulva with safe cleansing agent and water				
- uses downward strokes in cleansing				
- discards each swab after use				
- gives fluids throughout labour				

*"Plus" can mean either "yes" or "satisfactory". "Minus" can mean either "no"
or "unsatisfactory". "N.O." means "not observed".

	Performance			Comment
	Plus*	Minus*	N.O.*	
C. Care to mother in labour				
Provides appropriate care during labour				
- provides backrub for comfort				
- helps mother to change position as necessary				
- provides emotional support to mother				
- relates to family members in culturally prescribed manner				
- avoids unnecessary interference with birth process such as				
- strong massage of abdomen				
- insertion of hands into birth canal				
- administration of medications				
D. Recognition of normal progress during birth				
1. Palpates abdomen to determine				
- baby's position				
- quality and duration of contractions				
2. Observes perineum for abnormal bleeding				
3. Recognizes danger signs during labour				
- prolonged labour				
- convulsions during labour				
- breech or shoulder presentation of baby				
- prolapsed cord				
4. Responds appropriately to complications of delivery				
- summons midwife or physician if possible				
- initiates appropriate care until help arrives				
E. Performance of safe, hygienic delivery				
1. Prepares for delivery				
- puts on clean apron				
- thoroughly scrubs hands				
- watches perineum for appearance of baby's head				
2. Prevents perineal laceration				
- applies gentle pressure to baby's head to slow the delivery				
- instructs mother to pant so as to reduce speed of delivery of head				
- applies gentle manual support to perineal area				

	Performance			Comment
	Plus*	Minus*	N.O.*	
3. Delivers the baby				
- supports the head as it emerges				
- feels around baby's neck for cord				
- gently slips cord over head if it was found around neck				
- removes sac from head if it is present				
- wipes baby's eyes, nose, and mouth with clean swab as soon as head emerges				
- supports baby as its body emerges				
- inverts baby to drain mucus				
- places baby on clean cover between mother's legs				
4. Attends to umbilical cord				
- washes hands before manipulating cord				
- tests cord for cessation of pulsations				
- avoids contamination of cord ties				
- applies clean cord ties				
- ties square knots in applying cord ties				
- checks knots for security				
- lifts scissors by handles, avoiding contact with blades				
- cuts cord between the two cord ties				
- observes cord stump for bleeding				
- touches only edges of cord dressing				
- applies dressing, with cord in "turned up" position				
- avoids unsafe practices in cord care such as application of unclean materials, earth, saliva, ashes				
5. Prevents haemorrhage				
- puts baby to mother's breast to stimulate uterine contraction				
- identifies separation of placenta by watching for small gush of blood from birth canal				
- avoids pulling on placenta or membranes as placenta emerges				
- catches placenta in basin				
- inspects placenta carefully to see if it is complete				
- examines placenta for evidence of foul odour				
- inspects external genitals for fresh bleeding or lacerations				
- palpates uterine fundus frequently for hardness				
- massages uterus gently to control excessive blood loss				
- avoids unsafe practices such as packing birth canal to stop bleeding				

	Performance			Comment
	Plus*	Minus*	N.O.*	
F. After-care of mother				
Promotes mother's comfort after delivery				
- wipes perineum with clean swabs				
- uses downward strokes in wiping perineum				
- sponges mother				
- changes mother's clothing				
- provides clean mat to lie on				
- applies clean pad to perineum				
- offers food and drink				
- provides opportunity for rest				